The Take-Charge Patient

How YOU Can Get the Best Medical Care

Martine Ehrenclou, M.A.

LEMON
GROVE
PRESS

The Take-Charge Patient: How You Can Get The Best Medical Care
By Martine Ehrenclou, M.A.

Lemon Grove Press, LLC
1158 26th Street
Suite #502
Santa Monica, CA 90403

Fax: (310) 476-7627

www.TheTakeChargePatient.com
info@lemongrovepress.com

ISBN: 978-0-9815240-3-0

Library of Congress Control number: 2011913236

First Edition: Printed in the United States of America
0 9 8 7 6 5 4 3 2 1

Cover Design: George Foster

Interior Design and Layout: Sue Knopf

AUTHOR'S NOTE

The information in this book is not intended to substitute for medical or legal advice. The purpose is to inform readers by providing an overview of information available to assist patients and their loved ones to get the best medical care. It is not meant to contradict, disregard or interfere with any medical advice or medical care provided by medical professionals.

Every effort has been made to make this book as complete and accurate as possible based on the information available at the time of publication. The accuracy of the contents may change over time. Therefore, this text should be used as a general guide and not as the ultimate source of information.

In some instances, the names of individuals or institutions have been changed to protect privacy.

For Jamie, Lucy and Logan

Contents

Foreword

When Martine came to see me, she was similar to most of my patients: years of suffering from abdominal pain with no explanation, no diagnosis, and thus no treatment. She had sought the expertise of specialist after specialist, yet could not understand why no one had figured out the cause of her pain. To me, she was yet another patient with a fairly straightforward problem who needed a physician to listen to and truly hear her whole story.

I believe the most valuable quality of a physician today is his/her ability to listen. At the same time, the patient must do whatever it takes to capture the attention of their physician. In *The Take-Charge Patient*, Martine Ehrenclou provides tips and tricks needed to teach patients how to do exactly that. Chapter One starts with the quote from Osler, a revered medical educator, that I always share with my medical students, "Listen to the patient: he is telling you the diagnosis." In medical school, students are encouraged to sit down with the patient for a couple of hours and perform a thorough history and physical. By the time physicians are in practice, the history and physical becomes more focused, and multiple forces compel them to decrease their time with patients, thus reducing their attention to details. It is at this point that the role of the patient becomes so vital in assuring the quality of their care. *The Take-Charge Patient* is their reference guide to do so.

In her book, Martine preaches what she practices. The book is filled with a comprehensive and logically organized list of to-dos for patients. When I read it, my first thought was: "Wow, someone actually put all of my tips and tricks on how to navigate the medical system into a book."

My second thought was: "How in the heck did a nonmedical person have enough insight to write this book?"

As an academic surgeon with connections throughout the nation, I often have friends and family seek my input in their medical care. I refer them to physicians who are up to date in their field, technically skilled, well read, and most important, good listeners. If they can't get an appointment in a reasonable time, there are always options: a) find another equally qualified doctor, or b) be patient but persistent and put yourself on a cancellation wait list.

These principles as well as hundreds more useful tips are carefully listed in *The Take-Charge Patient*. The advice provided in this book is invaluable. Most patients are not aware of these details; however, in my experience, those patients of mine who have the most successful outcomes typically follow the advice outlined in this book:

- They do research about their symptoms.
- They carefully gather their medical records before the visit.
- They send their information ahead of their appointment.
- They include a short summary of their problems.
- They come prepared with a list of questions.
- They arrive with a partner who can also listen for them.
- If they have unanswered questions after their initial visit, they make a follow-up appointment.
- They are respectful of their physician, the staff and other healthcare providers.

Martine sent me her records and followed up with questions. She did her research. She was respectful of my time, and at the same time she took charge of her care. I, in turn, listened to Martine and helped alleviate her problem. She is now pain-free and the author of a book that I have already shared with my own family and that I will share with my patients, medical students, residents, and fellows in training.

Shirin Towfigh, MD, FACS
Associate Professor of Surgery
Hernia and Laparoscopic Specialist
Department of Surgery
Cedars-Sinai Medical Center
Los Angeles, California

Introduction

I began my journey into advocacy eleven years ago when my mother and godmother were patients in hospitals for very lengthy stays. I was not prepared for what I saw and experienced with their care. Hospitals were foreign worlds to me back then but I eventually learned the ropes and how to work the hospital system for their benefit.

I did not know at the time that what I was doing was called "advocacy." I simply thought I was helping my loved ones who were subjected to terrible neglect, misdiagnoses, medication mistakes and a variety of serious medical errors. It was their suffering at the hands of a system I once thought was the safest place a patient could be that drove me into the role of advocate and to write my award-winning book, *Critical Conditions: The Essential Hospital Guide to Get Your Loved One Out Alive.*

In August of 2009, I began interviews with more than 200 physicians and patients for a new book I was writing, *The Take-Charge Patient: How You Can Get the Best Medical Care.* This book was born out of my need to empower patients to become proactive, assertive and well-informed participants in their health care.

Six months into my research and interviews, I developed excruciating pelvic pain. Little did I know back in January of 2010 that I would go from author and advocate for others to advocate for myself using every single strategy in this book. It was an unexpected and ironic experiment to test what I had researched and learned from preeminent physicians, other medical professionals and patients from all over the country.

Over a period of sixteen months I became a take-charge patient. I consulted with twelve physicians of differing specialties and three alternative medicine practitioners and was given eleven diagnoses, twenty-two medications and fifteen procedures and surgeries to treat and cure my pain. It was not an easy journey for over a year and the pain compromised my life in a way I still have a hard time coming to terms with. But the end to the story is a happy one because my strategies in this book did in fact lead me to the right doctor who gave me the correct tests, diagnosis and treatment plan.

I am now pain free.

I never expected to live each chapter of this book, but it did prove to me just how invaluable this information is.

The Take-Charge Patient is about how to become your own advocate and get the best medical care for you. It focuses on teaching you to become a proactive and organized patient who is prepared to successfully navigate today's confusing and complicated health care system.

For *The Take-Charge Patient*, I interviewed more than 200 physicians, nurses, pharmacists, health psychologists, medical office managers, medical billers, patients and more. This book contains information straight from these medical professionals and patients as well as from hundreds of hours of my own research. It also contains information from my own medical journey, insights and strategies that no one taught me and that I figured out myself.

You will be given insider information to navigate the health care system with confidence and tips to cut through the red tape of any medical encounter. You will learn how to be in charge of your medical care, and as a by-product, you will feel more empowered as a patient. You'll become a skilled patient who knows how to get what she needs rather than a patient who is the recipient of what the health care system offers.

> "The more prepared a patient is, the more productive the office visit will be."
>
> Jack C. Rosenfeld, MD, Family Medicine and Geriatrics, Lansdale, PA

You'll acquire strategies to beat a system that at times seems bound and determined to beat you.

By learning how to advocate for yourself as a patient, you'll be part of the act instead of part of the audience.

Taking charge of yourself as a patient is essential in order for your doctors and other medical professionals to serve you in the way they know best. After reading this book, you will be in a position to get medical care anywhere in the world. You will have all of your necessary medical information in your possession so that you can prevent what we've all experienced: scrambling to gather our information from a variety of sources who aren't necessarily making you their first priority. You'll learn how to find the best doctor for you, collaborate and effectively communicate with that doctor, prepare for medical appointments, do credible research, prevent medical errors and medication mistakes, find discounted or free medical care and medications, and much more. You'll learn how to manage your health insurance, something most of us just dread doing and have trouble understanding.

> "If you're proactive in your medical care, then I'll be more proactive. I'll be more involved because you've shown a vested interest."
>
> Linda Nadwodny, DO, FAAFP, Family Medicine, Lansdale, PA

Your health care is a team sport. By being proactive, involved and organized, you'll find that your medical professionals will respond to you more positively and with more respect.

SPECIAL NOTE: If you read this book from cover to cover, you will note that some information is repeated in separate chapters. I purposely repeated important information so that nothing would be missed by those readers who only read certain chapters.

For the sake of grammatical simplicity, I have used the pronouns *she* and *her* throughout the book; however, the information is equally valuable for men.

1

How I Became a Take-Charge Patient

*"Listen to the patient. He is telling you
the diagnosis."*

SIR WILLIAM OSLER, FATHER OF MODERN MEDICINE

It was the first week of January 2010. I was working on my new book, *The Take-Charge Patient*, wrapping up six months of interviews with physicians, nurses, pharmacists, patients and more. I was excited by the information I had learned from my research, from esteemed medical professionals and patients from all over the country.

I knew I was onto something with my new book. I remember telling a friend that the writing was going so well that I thought that I might have the first draft completed in six months.

Little did I know that within two weeks I would develop debilitating pelvic pain that would last for over a year and that my life would be severely compromised in ways I could never have imagined. Unbeknownst to me that first week of January, I would end up using every strategy in my new book and living every single chapter to become a take-charge patient.

During those sixteen months, I saw twelve doctors, many of differing specialties, plus three alternative medicine practitioners, in an effort to figure out what was wrong with me and end my pain. I was given eleven diagnoses, was prescribed twenty-two medications, and endured fifteen procedures and surgeries. The pain was simply indescribable. A few times I wondered just how much more I could take.

It was the third week of January. I was recovering from a nasty chest cold. I rose out of bed one morning, still coughing as I had the night before. I don't remember exactly when the pelvic pain began that day. Pain has a way of muddling our thoughts and memories. I do remember feeling pain in that area during my dance class, wondering at the time what it was, brushing it off to a possible bladder infection.

Days later I was in my gynecologist's office, undergoing tests. This began the onslaught of misdiagnoses, multiple antibiotics, tests, procedures, injections and surgeries.

My journey began with a misdiagnosis of interstitial cystitis (IC), a lifelong condition for which there is no cure. After doing research and discovering that I did not have two of the five major symptoms, I started to doubt the diagnosis.

It wasn't easy doubting a physician I'd known and liked for many years. I wanted to believe her, partly because she has education, training and a medical degree but also because I trusted her. To test out her theory, I did abide by the IC diet that withheld acid-producing foods and liquids. Nothing reduced my pain.

After two weeks of experimenting with the IC diet, I went to a urologist for a second opinion. He rejected my gynecologist's diagnosis of IC and offered his own, plus multiple rounds of antibiotics and some pain medication. After three months of painful exams, bladder procedures and tests, I was no better off than I was in January. The pain persisted and grew worse, stifling my participation in family outings, dance classes, work and more.

I sought a third opinion from another urologist. He did an exam and a set of tests and found nothing to warrant antibiotics. He instructed me to stop taking the antibiotics I'd been given and to eat a macrobiotic diet. This was the third conflicting medical opinion. Which was I to choose?

Frustrated that all three physicians had disagreed with one another, I became my own medical detective in search of a diagnosis. I sought more opinions from other specialists. The first was a highly respected gynecologist who specializes in fibroids because I wanted to find out if fibroids were the cause of my problem. They weren't.

I then consulted with my internist whom I'd known for twenty years. I asked his advice. He talked to the other specialists I'd seen and reviewed their theories. He explained that I had differing opinions from very respected doctors. Still no accurate diagnosis.

The pain wore on and my drive increased to find a correct diagnosis that would end my pain. I soon realized that I had been using many of the strategies in my own book. I was becoming a take-charge patient. For each medical encounter, I arrived prepared with copies of my medical records, list of medications, health summary, test results, lists of doctors I'd seen and what they had diagnosed me with. I kept a notebook with me at all times and recorded my symptoms, when they occurred and what made them worse or better. I researched every doctor I saw, every diagnosis, each treatment plan, every medication, and I discussed my findings with my husband and close friends, fishing for information and ideas as we talked.

By August of 2010, I was unable to complete a dance class without pain erupting with terrific force, unable to sit at my desk for more than a half hour before pain gripped me from beneath, tugging and twisting my insides. I continued as my own advocate, with the help of my husband and a couple of close friends.

Since I had no success with traditional doctors, I decided to try the alternative medicine route. I figured two highly respected acupuncturists/ Chinese herbalists would be able to help me. After ingesting smelly teas and enduring hours of needles stuck in my arms, legs and face, I still was no closer to relief from the pain or to a diagnosis.

By November of 2010, I began losing steam. I was worn down, discouraged and fatigued by ongoing pain. I was becoming isolated; I avoided friends, turned down all social invitations and missed out on time with my family. My ability to work slowed. My dance classes were a thing of the past and my afternoons were spent lying down after a day of trying to forge on.

It's funny how chronic pain has a way of absorbing your life. At first you summon your energy to get multiple opinions to find an answer, do your own research, and discuss your findings with loved ones. Every effort is channeled into presenting yourself to doctors as a patient who is professional and worthy of respect—one to be taken seriously. But when every treatment, test, procedure, medication and diagnosis fails, you are left with yourself and your body. Chronic pain is a lonely business. The sense of isolation and loneliness I felt was simply indescribable. The fear that I would never get better was with me most of the time, draining my energy, my hope and my confidence in doctors.

I now only discussed my medical condition with my husband and a couple of close friends. To the rest of the world, I pretended I was fine. I faked it to most, not wanting outside interference or having to explain one more time why I wasn't getting better.

It was at this time that a good friend of mine, who is very medically savvy, became much more involved in helping me. She agreed to be my advocate and offered continuous support and encouragement. F. researched my symptoms, possible diagnoses and current diagnoses I'd been given by physicians. We discussed everything we both uncovered on a regular basis. We brainstormed possible steps for me to take. F. grew more and more invested in helping me find the right doctor and the right tests to determine what was causing me such pain. She accompanied me to some appointments with new doctors and we discussed what had transpired in the office visits.

In this book and in my last, I have written about the importance of enlisting a loved one to be a patient's advocate. The impact of just how important that really is hit me when I realized I could no longer handle everything myself. My husband comforted me and discussed my symptoms with me—he listened to me ad nauseam when I shared ideas. He even came up with ideas of his own. F. and I shared research and ideas, brainstorming regularly. Another close friend offered consistent support and comfort. I can never thank my husband and F. and my other friends enough for their faith that I was going to get better and find the reason for my chronic pelvic pain. I had a good support system.

One day, F. brought up the fact that I'd had four abdominal surgeries over my lifetime and suggested that adhesions or scar tissue could be the cause of my pain. She suggested that I consult a surgeon. I did.

After faxing my medical records and health summary to the surgeon who had performed one of my surgeries, we talked on the phone. He said he didn't believe there was any chance that there could be complications such as adhesions. He said he would be happy to see me in an office visit and recommended that I see a gastroenterologist.

I did take his suggestion and made an appointment for an overdue colonoscopy in hopes that something might be uncovered with that test. But I just didn't buy this surgeon's opinion that no complications could have arisen after four abdominal surgeries. F. and I discussed which medical professional to see next.

We asked ourselves which tests could determine adhesions, scar tissue or other issues that might have resulted from my C-section, belly button hernia repair from my pregnancy, gall bladder surgery and abdominal liposuction some twenty years ago. Who better to ask these questions of than a radiologist who specializes in imaging tests?

I called a radiologist I knew. After faxing my medical records, including test results, health summary, health history, list of doctors I'd seen and my previous diagnoses, I asked him which tests could reveal any aftereffects of my four abdominal surgeries. I explained my medical condition and the idea of adhesions or scar tissue as possible causes of my pain. This doctor said, "There is no test that can reveal scar tissue, adhesions or what you are looking for. Stick to the doctors you're working with. They know what they are doing." There was no point in explaining that I was simply looking for a clue to my next step, not going behind any doctor's back.

I thought a lot about what this radiologist had said. A couple of other doctors I'd seen for second opinions had also suggested that I stick with the doctor I was working with. I realized then that some doctors are in close-knit communities and watch each other's backs, protecting each other even at the expense of the patient. I've heard from other medical professionals that this kind of loyalty is based on friendships, mutual referrals and a sense of protectiveness of one another. Perhaps fear of being sued also factors into the equation.

I still didn't give up. I knew persistence was key to finding the right doctor, the right diagnosis and the right treatment plan. With the support of my husband, my medically savvy friend, F., and a couple of other close friends, I pushed forward.

One day my husband came home and shared a suggestion from a friend of his. "M. said you should go see the urogynecologist his wife sees." The next day F. suggested the very same doctor.

By the time I entered Dr. R.'s office in December of 2010, amost a year after my pain began, I was weak, vulnerable and exhausted. I presented this doctor with ten pages of my health history. Seated at her desk, she read every word. After a few pages she motioned to my health history and records and said, "This is very helpful. Thank you."

As she read, I thought about the upcoming holidays. I dreaded them. We had family coming in from out of town and a ski vacation planned. I knew I was not up for either.

Still reading, Dr. R. said, "You poor thing." Her empathy meant more to me than I could possibly express. I suspected she knew what kind of pain I'd been experiencing. I thought about the painful urological procedures I'd undergone, how after they were over I'd left the urologist's office only to slide into my car, call my husband and cry while still in the medical building parking lot.

This was the first time a doctor other than my internist had expressed empathy. Kind, caring and smart, Dr. R. reassured me that she would help me. She said it might take time but that she would do everything she could. I could have hugged her.

The holidays passed and I missed my family's ski trip, avoided all holiday parties, and while family visited us, I spent a lot of time in bed. I went through with the colonoscopy in early January and was disappointed when the results yielded nothing. No one wants something to be wrong unless she's suffered with ongoing pain or discomfort with no diagnosis or cure.

Around the middle of January, Dr. R. ordered tests, including a pelvic ultrasound, to rule out serious medical issues. One friend said to me, "You mean to tell me you haven't had a pelvic ultrasound yet with all the doctors you've seen?" At least Dr. R. was on top of things. She prescribed non-narcotic pain medications and asked me to report in to her. She returned my phone calls and emails. When she asked me to do something, I did it. When I brought up questions and shared the research I'd done, she listened and discussed what I had found. When I asked her if endometriosis could be causing the pain, she did tests to find out. She didn't brush me off—she respected me as her patient.

Even though Dr. R. was the medical expert, we had a collaborative working relationship. Our doctor-patient relationship was based on trust.

I knew she was an excellent doctor and I suspect she knew I was a credible reporter on my body.

On my third office visit with her, she tried something new. She asked me to bear with her for a moment while she pressed on trigger points in my pelvic region. She asked which were tender or painful. She said, "Let's try something." She injected an anesthetic into my pelvic nerves and then asked me to engage in the activities that brought on the most pain. I raced to my office and sat at my desk.

There was no pain.

I called Dr. R.'s office and her staff was almost as giddy as I was.

This began two and a half months of biweekly injections of an anesthetic and steroid into my pelvic nerves. As painful as these injections were, most of the time they were successful. Some numbed the pain for a few days, others not at all. But they gave me hope for a cure. Dr. R. gave me hope. She was the first doctor who thought outside of her specialty, who thought outside of the box. For the first time in a year, I had many days when I was actually able to sit at my desk for short periods of time and get through part of a dance class.

But it didn't last.

Dr. R. told me I needed to see a specialist who could do more for me, someone who specialized in treating this kind of pelvic pain. The thought of seeing yet another doctor when I had hinged my hopes on her was simply unthinkable. Dr. R. explained that the injections were not eradicating my pain in a permanent way as she had hoped.

My hope plummeted. Back to square one. I didn't want to see another doctor, especially after finally finding one who really wanted to help me, who used her own time to do research on my case and who talked to other doctors about my medical condition and possible treatments.

Accompanied by my medically savvy friend, I then saw a pelvic pain specialist. Even though I had researched him ahead of time and found impressive credentials, I was suspect from the onset. He rented an exam room in a big medical practice and required payment in cash.

Dr. A. was not interested in my medical history, list of medications or health summary. He didn't look me in the eye. He rushed through the first five minutes of my office visit and asked me to get up on the exam table.

He asked his nurse to prepare some sort of injection. He then focused on locating trigger points. He whipped out a syringe and needle the length of a ruler. I had to stop him. I said, "Wait please." I asked him what he thought my diagnosis was, asked him what his treatment plan was, and what he was about to do. He took the time to explain but I could tell he was not used to patients like me.

After his explanation, he gave me injections and told me to come back at the same time next week. He handed me a prescription for pain medication without knowing which medications I was already taking. I never filled it.

I gave Dr. A. another chance only because I was desperate. His credentials were good, so I held on to false hope and made excuses for his behavior. The next time I saw him, he did not remember where he had last injected me and when I showed him, he asked me why he had injected me so high up on my abdomen. Maybe it was because I was so tired, in pain, and not thinking clearly, but I allowed him to inject me again. Nothing he did relieved my pain. Not only was I out a sizeable amount of cash, but I was also no better off. I never went back.

My next step was to see a highly respected neurologist. I did my usual research on this doctor before I saw him, called a couple of doctors I'd interviewed for this book and asked for their opinions about him. Each comment was more glowing than the last. Dr. Z. believed my pelvic pain originated in my lower back. He said he could perform a surgical procedure that would relieve the pain.

What Dr. Z. explained made sense to me at the time. But when I arrived at the surgery center, I had a bad feeling. Parked outside of the surgery center at 6 o'clock on a Wednesday morning, my anxiety mounted. I started an argument with my husband, all because I was so nervous and couldn't put my finger on the source of my worry. I went ahead with the procedure. I was anesthetized and then awakened while needles in my lower back were electrically stimulated to elicit a response in my pelvic region and then steroids were injected. The procedure didn't work.

This was the end of the line for me.

I plunged into depression. After seeing so many doctors plus three alternative medicine professionals, trying so many medications and just about everything else, I had had enough. I thought about all the people who cope with some form of chronic pain with no understanding of its root cause—only treatment for the symptoms. I was terrified that this was going to be my future.

In early May of 2011, I was researching "hiatal hernia" for a good friend of mine who had just been diagnosed with it. As I searched on the internet, I spotted an article in a highly respected newspaper. The headline read, "In women, hernias can be hidden agony." I knew my friend had been dealing with some discomfort so I began reading. The third line talked about pelvic pain. It was a story about a woman who had agonizing pelvic pain and the root cause was hidden hernias with fat protruding through the holes, pressing on nerves.

My heart raced as I read the article. The woman described was just like me with the same symptoms. My instinct told me that this was my problem. I just knew it. I read that article twice and discovered that the surgeon, who specialized in hernias, was located in Los Angeles at a major teaching hospital that was affiliated with a highly respected medical school.

My hands shook as I called the surgeon's office and made an appointment.

I called my medically savvy friend, my husband and a couple of other friends and sent them the link to the article. Whether they believed it or not, each person supported me and my conviction that this was, in fact, it.

Dr. T. was lovely. During my examination, she told me she thought I had hernias and ordered a high-resolution dynamic MRI.

The MRI showed that I had a muscle tear at my C-section site, an inguinal hernia, and a belly-button hernia. I was elated when Dr. T. gave me the results. I hoped this would be the end to sixteen long months of pelvic pain.

Until I interviewed ministers, rabbis and other religious professionals for a chapter in this book, I had no idea what they offered to people who have medical problems, surgeries, hospitalizations and more. I had been calling our church's prayer line for many months, asking them to pray for an accurate diagnosis, a treatment plan and the right doctor to execute both. This time I called and asked for prayer for my surgery and its success. I then received a call from our minister and associate minister, both offering their support and a visit after my surgery. Then I received phone calls from our church deacons to see if I needed anything, such as meals. I was so touched by all of their gestures. I thought back to my chapter about how religious institutions help people in medical need. Again, I was living out one of my book's chapters and realizing its value.

I had surgery two weeks later to repair the muscle tear and the hernias. My surgeon explained that in addition to the muscle tear, I also had an inguinal hernia with a nerve that passed through the hole and got pinched every time I exercised, walked, sat in a chair, rode in a car or hunched over. This had caused the excruciating pain.

Thankfully, the surgery was successful and I am now pain free.

To say that I am grateful to Dr. T. is an understatement. She gave me my life back. She is exactly the kind of doctor I recommend in this book if you need a highly trained specialist. She was

- affiliated with a highly respected medical school;

- very experienced with the kind of surgery I was about to have;

- nice and caring.

The fact that she performed my surgery on a Saturday morning because she was leaving the country shortly thereafter tells you a lot about her.

I am also very grateful to Dr. R., my urogynecologist, who took such good care of me and showed me exactly what a doctor-patient relationship should be, just as I describe it in this book. She taught me by example and experience what every single doctor I interviewed for this book told me:

Find a doctor:

- who you like;

- who you can talk to and who listens to you;

- who you can collaborate with in a partnership;

- who respects you;

- who will reach out to other physicians for more information, putting ego aside;

- who returns phone calls;

- who is invested in your health and well-being.

I now have my life back. I consider myself to be incredibly lucky and now well versed in my own strategies. I've implemented them, tried them out firsthand and realize their value.

A take-charge patient needs the strategies in this book, but she also needs persistence. Persistence is the key to finding solutions to both simple and complex medical issues. Even if you are healthy, you need persistence to get the kind of medical care you deserve. I hope this book helps every single one of you.

2

How You Become a Take-Charge Patient

*"Patients who are proactive
get much better medical care."*

ZOUHDI A. HAJJAJ, MD,
INTERNAL MEDICINE, YARMOUTHPORT, MA

If you go to a car mechanic, you know something's wrong with your car but you may not know the cause. You describe in detail how it rattles, how the engine turns over or how the air conditioning doesn't work. You are armed with information for the professional who is going to fix your car.

We don't always do that with physicians. Often we go to the doctor thinking she will ask all the right questions, will have our current list of medications at her fingertips, will remember exactly why we were seen six months ago, will recall the conversation we had with her on the phone about a new medication that we had stopped, and will instantly summon all she needs to know about us as soon as she enters the exam room and opens our chart.

Wrong.

Most doctors are breaking their necks to see as many patients as they can, both to accommodate patients and to pay the bills. Not an easy job when their reimbursements from health insurance companies steadily decrease each year and their office overhead rapidly increases. Doctors must keep up with technology, educate themselves about the many new drugs that regularly come on the market, talk to specialists who see their patients, see patients in their offices, visit patients in hospitals, do mountains of paperwork demanded by insurance companies on each and every patient, haggle with health insurance companies over covering treatments, medications and procedures they know their patients need, and much more.

The days of doctors making a lot of money and spending Wednesday afternoons on the golf course are gone.

It's time for us to step up to the plate and take charge of ourselves as patients. Not because all doctors are falling down on their jobs (although some are) but because most doctors no longer can function in the way they once did in the time of Marcus Welby. And neither can we as patients. The health care system has changed radically and has become increasingly complicated. Forty years ago doctors made house calls and many patients had only one doctor who managed their medical care. Doctors didn't have health insurance companies to haggle with over their patients' medical treatments. If a doctor wants to stay afloat today, she must compromise in ways she might not feel comfortable with.

You are a big part of getting excellent medical care from your doctor or other medical professional. Your doctor cannot do her work without your input. It simply doesn't work any more to be a passive patient who sits back and waits for the doctor to take care of everything.

"My successful patients are well informed, knowledgeable about their conditions, the options open to them. They know the medicines that are available. This jump-starts the whole process and makes the whole interaction more efficient and satisfying for all parties involved."

Daniel Wohlgelernter, MD,
Cardiology, Santa Monica, CA

I interviewed several doctors who are considering getting out of the profession because they simply cannot do the job they aspire to. One anonymous doctor said, "My life is miserable now. I decided I made a mistake and think I should have been a veterinarian." When I asked him why, he said, "The administrative burden of medicine has become horrible. The ultimate goal today is to reduce the cost of medicine. That I understand. But when I have nonmedical professionals in certain insurance companies tying my hands by telling me I have to use certain medications and I may not feel those are the right medications for my patients, that's where I draw the line."

We can't change the health care system or the way doctors practice medicine, but we can change how we as patients approach the two. And changing our approach is essential to getting what we want and need from our medical care.

It's time to change our experience as patients.

Prepare for Your Doctor's Appointment

If we gear up for appointments with our doctors the way we gear up for meetings with attorneys or tax accountants, we approach them with confidence and preparation. We are in charge even though we are going to them for advice and with the faith that they will help solve our problem. It's been too easy for us to see doctors and assume they will take care of everything and that we don't have to

> "Patients need to feel they have more control over their medical care."
>
> Jack C. Rosenfeld, MD, Family Medicine and Geriatrics, Lansdale, PA

do much but answer questions, be examined and listen to treatment plans or instructions. And too often we are dissatisfied with our medical care, mistrustful of our doctors and medications, confused about what is wrong with us and what we can do about it. As a result, we don't follow through with treatment plans and are angry about the care we received.

As patients, we need to empower ourselves not only for our own well-being, but also to ensure that our medical treatment is as successful as possible.

A take-charge patient can go anywhere in the world and get medical treatment because she has her medical history, complete health file, medical records, and a list of medications and allergies to medications at her disposal. She does not need to call any doctor or pharmacist to find out which drugs she is taking, which medical conditions she has, and which tests, surgeries or procedures she has undergone. She has it all in her possession.

With my chronic medical condition, each time I saw a new doctor, I came prepared with my medical records, copies of new test results, dates and reports on surgeries and procedures, a list of medications and allergies to medications and research. I had everything with me. I even had a short health summary prepared for each medical professional.

I can almost guarantee you that if you walk into a doctor's office with a prepared list of questions, prioritized according to importance, a brief health summary, and copies of your medical records, your doctor will take you more seriously. What results? Better medical care. Many doctors explained that a good relationship with your medical professional is an integral part of successful medical care.

You don't want to be like the patient I encountered when I was recently in a doctor's office. This patient was on her cell phone pacing up and down the hall, calling her pharmacy for a list of all the medications she was taking and calling her other doctor for the names of treatments and procedures she had undergone. I heard it all. I watched her pace, sensed her anxiety, sensed the pressure she was under to gather all the information to present to her new doctor. I felt sorry for her, wanted to tell her what to do in the future because there are solutions to the problems she was having.

Relying on someone who knows so much more about how our bodies work than we do takes a leap of faith. It takes a much shorter leap to trust our doctors if we understand what our diagnosis is, why the doctor thinks the diagnosis is correct, what is proposed to treat us and why. Many studies confirm that if a patient is involved in this way, she will be much more apt to follow the physician's recommendations and will get better faster and more easily.

Take Charge of What You Can

If we want the kind of medical care that feels worth the money, then we are simply going to have to take some responsibility and do some of the work ourselves. Take-charge patients are proactive and assertive without being belligerent and overly demanding. We ask questions when we need to, and we treat our doctors with respect and expect the same in return. Even if we are afraid to ask questions because we think the doctor will get annoyed, we ask anyway, because it is our health we are talking about, not a car. If a car isn't fixed properly, we can use another form of transportation. If our health isn't good, we don't have alternatives. We need our health to lead fulfilling lives, to take care of our children, to be productive at work and to take care of our families and our homes. Without good health, we have nothing.

I know. I lost good health for sixteen months. I felt dependent on the doctors who were treating me because I could not diagnose or treat myself. But I trusted my instincts, educated myself, enlisted help from loved ones and organized my health records. I learned how to interact with doctors as an assertive, educated and informed patient while still being amiable and respectful. I was persistent. For sixteen months I kept going, kept pursuing answers, dialogued with doctors about possible diagnoses and solutions to my medical condition. I persisted with my research and simply refused to give up.

Not that I didn't question myself along the way, question the doctors, fall back in frustration because for so long I was not getting better. There were times I wanted to give up. There were times during my diagnosis journey that the ongoing pain and frustration were just too much. I am so grateful for a supportive husband and good friends. They all helped me at crucial times to get reinvested in my health.

Invest in Your Health

If you are disinterested in your health, don't care enough to become proactive in your medical care, don't do what the doctor says, forget appointments, don't follow through with your doctor's medical advice and don't communicate with her about it, I can almost promise you that your medical care will be compromised. Not because the doctor wants it that way. We do what is necessary to get the best medical care possible.

"A patient must understand why a medical treatment was suggested. This increases compliance greatly. Patients are more inclined to do lifestyle changes when they understand the reasons behind the doctor's suggestions and recommendations."

Frank Sievert, MD,
Family Medicine, Corvallis, OR

"I had a cardiomyopathy patient. He was a dockworker. He was 38 when he started to have trouble with shortness of breath. He could not unload the ship as he had in the past. The patient had a severe systolic cardiomyopathy (severe heart failure) from hepatitis C. His tests showed that his heart was only able to perform at less than 50% normal. After he became a self-

advocate, he gave up drinking and some other bad habits. His heart function improved 40% over two years time. He started calling me and checking in about worsened symptoms prior to the issues becoming severe. He became more proactive. I told him what to do and then asked him to call me back. He did it. At the end of a couple of years of positive interaction, he got quite a bit better. He was able to operate the top pick on the docks, drive, and help his wife with cleaning the house and walking the dog. This degree of improvement is very rare with his condition. Unfortunately, the story did not have a happy ending. He finally lost his battle against his illness after seven years' time."

Alan Bailer, DO, Internal Medicine, Cheltenham, PA

> "Patients deny they have the symptoms because they don't want to be sick or to admit anything is wrong."
>
> Alan Jasper, MD,
> Internal Medicine
> and Pulmonary Diseases,
> Los Angeles, CA

Many of us think we are never going to get sick. Think again. Many of us think we are invincible until something goes wrong.

People may call take-charge patients control freaks, but who would you want as your advocate when you are in serious medical need—a take-charge patient or someone who goes with the flow?

Asked and answered.

Be Assertive

Take-charge patients are assertive and persistent. We don't act this way to be obnoxious, although sometimes we are. We call a doctor's office every week to grab an unexpected cancellation when the doctor isn't scheduled to see us for two months. We get second opinions on our medical conditions.

"In February 1996, my mom called me from New York with the news that she had been diagnosed with breast cancer. It had already spread to other parts of her body and the prognosis was not good. She rarely had checkups and had been healthy her whole life—ate well, never smoked or drank, etc.

I decided to have a mammogram, as I knew that breast cancer runs in families. Armed with the info about my mother,

I visited my OB/GYN and got a checkup and referral for a mammogram. My mammogram was clear and no lumps were found. Three months later, I found a dime-sized lump in my armpit at the "tail" of the breast. I was immediately sent to a surgeon for a lumpectomy and node biopsy. It was malignant and classed as a very aggressive type. Out of twelve nodes, seven tested positive for cancer cells. I was given an aggressive form of chemotherapy, followed by radiation. I was given the prognosis of a 60% chance of reoccurrence. Not good odds.

When I first sought treatment, I was told that, given the size of my lump, the cancer had been growing for at least three years. I do not have much faith in mammograms but get one yearly along with a breast MRI every two years for good measure. I have been cancer free ever since."

Gail, Patient, Santa Monica, CA

Gail is a perfect example of a take-charge patient. Even though her mammograms were clear, she was not complacent. She did breast exams and when she found a lump, she did something about it.

Be Persistent

Take-charge patients are persistent but not belligerent or hostile. We are firm and respectful. When we have not received test results, we call the doctor and ask for them. When we don't understand something the doctor has said, we ask for clarification. We research suggested medications and treatment plans to make sure they are right for us and so we can have more effective conversations with our doctors. We get second and third opinions until a diagnosis feels right. We may be embarrassed over not understanding medical jargon but we ask the doctor to explain the terms she is using anyway. We do not put up with doctors treating us like children and, in turn, we do not treat our doctors like parents.

Be Charming and Polite

Take-charge patients are also charming and polite. Ever get a table at a jam-packed restaurant because you charmed the host? Charm the hosts! If you are friendly and appreciative, most of your medical professionals will find it much easier to help you. Even when you aren't feeling well, the trick is to remain diplomatic when your doctor's front office person is acting cranky.

Only yesterday I called a doctor's office and asked about a $2,500 pathology bill from a procedure that my health insurance didn't cover. The front desk person was aloof and cavalier about the doctor using a pathology lab that charges that kind of money. I wanted to tell her a number of things at that moment, but I didn't. I reminded myself that I might need her in the future. I then called the pathology lab and asked for a discount. Unfortunately, my health insurance company had already interceded so a discount was out of the question. I then asked if I could make payments. The answer was yes.

Patients who are gracious and say thank you get better care. Why? Because they create amiable relationships with the medical professionals in their lives. They know that if they are ornery, the medical professionals will be less apt to want to engage. It's human nature.

It's a doctor's duty to help you as a patient but if you are nasty, you are only doing yourself a disservice. Nobody is motivated to help nasty people.

Have Reasonable Expectations

Even when we don't feel well, take-charge patients do not expect the doctor to do it all—we have reasonable expectations because we understand what today's doctors are up against. We also understand that doctors are not perfect and that medicine is not an exact science. As much as we want our doctors to be all-knowing, they simply are not. All the more reason to become a take-charge patient and do your research.

> "Allow for the fact that there is uncertainty in medicine."
>
> David B. Baron, MD,
> Family Medicine, Malibu, CA,
> Former Chief of Staff,
> Santa Monica-UCLA Medical
> Center & Orthopaedic Hospital

> "Work with the physician. Don't expect a miracle. Medicine is not a miracle. It is not a cookbook."
>
> Lynda Farrell, MD,
> Internal Medicine, Oakland, NJ

Many doctors said that patients expect them to be perfect, to know it all. We have to realize that doctors are not experienced in every aspect of medicine but that most are very educated and experienced in some or many areas.

As take-charge patients, we understand that doctors are not wizards and if we want to get better, we'd better do our part to support their efforts. That said, some doctors do believe they are gods. Those are the doctors with the "God complex" and we may need them at certain times in our lives, but may have a difficult time dealing with them. Those doctors perpetuate the myth that doctors have all-knowing powers and will magically heal us. It's time to change our perceptions of the medical professionals in our lives and see them as human beings with skills we need.

I went through unnecessary procedures, surgeries and medical treatments. I spent money I didn't have and took medications I didn't need, all because of misdiagnoses. Did I get mad? Yes. Was I frustrated? Yes. Was I disillusioned about doctors? Yes. But at the same time I also developed reasonable expectations of most physicians. I realized firsthand that I have to do some of the work myself to avoid any possible mishaps. I'm grateful when I find really good doctors.

It's About Confidence

When I talk to people about being take-charge patients, nearly every time one or two ask, "How can I ask a doctor to wash her hands before touching me?" They say that they are uncomfortable doing so because doctors are the bosses.

Not so.

Doctors are no more the bosses than you are. You work in partnership with your doctors. If you are frightened of speaking up (I've been there myself), then simply ask in a polite manner for the doctor to wash her hands. Make up an excuse about being worried about all the super bugs the media has been publicizing or say that you've become a little paranoid because you've been sick so much this winter.

"The blessing is that there are many medical professionals who have answers. The curse is that it is impossible and literally unethical for any medical professional to know the answers to everything. Because medicine is so specialized, it is impossible to know about all branches of medicine since it takes a lifetime just to learn one. Answering questions outside of one's specialty does a disservice to the patient, because there are other doctors who are specifically trained and experienced in handling these problems. This can be a source of frustration and terror for patients in the face of life-threatening conditions, when they are looking for answers from what they want to be an all knowing doctor."

Roger E. Dafter, PhD,
Associate Director,
Mind-Body Medicine Group,
Division of Head and Neck Surgery,
UCLA David Geffen School of
Medicine, Los Angeles, CA

I'll give you an example. I took my daughter to a pediatrician who was filling in for our regular pediatrician. We were in an exam room waiting for the doctor. Across the hall, I could see her in another exam room with two coughing children. She left there and walked straight into our room. I waited a few seconds for her to wash her hands as we exchanged pleasantries. She grabbed her stethoscope and approached my daughter. I said, "Would you mind washing your hands before touching my daughter? I'm sorry, but I know there are sick kids in this office." She hesitated for a second, her eye on me, and then turned toward the sink and washed her hands. Uncomfortable for a second? Yes, but it was worth it.

Being a take-charge patient means having confidence in yourself. It also means seeing your physician as an equal. Yes, they have degrees, training and experience that you don't but that doesn't mean you treat them as if they are bosses or parents. Doctors are people just like you and me, and if you treat them that way, you'll develop more confidence. Just by engaging in the behavior, even if you don't feel it at the time, the feeling will follow. It's like exercising a muscle.

Not that it isn't easy to slip into a submissive role when you are greeted by a physician with an authoritarian manner. I've done that myself. Even now, I sometimes clam up because I sense nonverbal cues from doctors who don't necessarily want me to participate in the delivery of my care. But I stop myself midway and summon my confidence.

How to Gain Confidence as a Take-Charge Patient

Here are a few tips on how to gain confidence with medical professionals:

- Gain control by organizing all of your medical records.
- Come prepared to a doctor's appointment with a list of questions and concerns, prioritized according to their importance to you.
- Educate yourself. Do research ahead of time on what you want to address with the doctor.
- Ask questions.
- Have copies of all your medical records in your possession.
- Be polite.

One of the main strategies for gaining confidence as a patient is to take control of what you can. If you come prepared for an office visit in anticipation of the doctor's questions, you won't be caught off guard. This means that you prepare a list of questions ahead of time, prioritize your top three medical concerns, take notes in a notebook on any symptoms you've been experiencing, create a health summary, and bring copies of medical records that are pertinent to the visit.

If you implement these steps, you will be more confident about what is happening with your medical care. Instead of allowing the doctor to take charge of everything and simply dole out advice, which puts you in a passive role, you educate yourself so you approach the doctor on an equal footing.

Besides, most doctors are no longer able to handle every detail for their patients. To some, it will be a relief that you have organized everything for them. To a few others, it might feel like you are usurping their control. But more on that in Chapter 5.

The more educated you are about your health and medical conditions from credible sources, the more empowered you will feel.

Almost every medical professional I interviewed said, "The single most important thing you can do is to be an active member of your health care team."

What to Do If Being a Take-Charge Patient Is Not Welcomed

It's fair to say that there are some doctors who don't want to see take-charge patients. For some medical professionals, it's easier to have the kind of doctor-patient relationship where the doctor simply tells the patient what to do and hopes she will do it.

Today's patients are much more educated and have access to more information than ever before.

However, there are still doctors who are used to their way of offering medical care or simply are too busy and overwhelmed to collaborate with a patient.

> "Most doctors will say they're open to proactive patients but at times it can make some uneasy."
>
> Roger E. Dafter, PhD,
> UCLA David Geffen
> School of Medicine,
> Los Angeles, CA

"I have three cancers and Alpha-1 (Antitrypsin Deficiency, an inherited emphysema that causes lung disease). I was about to have surgery to remove a malignant tumor from my prostate. I called the surgeon and asked a lot of questions. He got upset with me and said he had other patients waiting and he didn't have the time to take me through medical school. I enlisted help from my neighbors. They went with me to the surgeon's office. They helped me explain to him that I just wanted knowledge, wanted to know what was going to happen. That doctor treated me very differently after my neighbors talked to him. They helped me communicate with him and everything was fine after that."

John O. Will, Patient, Horsham, PA

What to Do If You Are Met with Resistance from a Doctor

- You can do what patient John O. Will did—enlist family or friends to help you communicate with your doctor. Meeting in person with an advocate is the best way to help change the dynamics with your doctor.

- Explain to your doctor that you want to be involved in your care, want to understand exactly what your diagnosis and treatment plan are so you can better comply with them. The word "comply" is a good buzzword to use with doctors. Many doctors complained about patients who don't "comply" with their treatment plans.

- You can make an appointment or simply ask your doctor when the best time is to talk about your upcoming procedure, surgery, treatment, etc.

- If, for example, you doubt your doctor's diagnosis and/or treatment plan, you can always say, "I know you're busy but I'm concerned about this. I need to ask you more questions." You might need to make another appointment for a short office visit.

- If the doctor is too busy to answer enough of your questions, ask if there is someone else in the office who could educate you on your upcoming procedure (such as a registered nurse, nurse practitioner or physician's assistant).

- Lastly, if your doctor simply is not interested in your collaboration, you might have to look for another doctor.

Patients who are involved get better medical care.

PATIENT CHECKLIST

Am I ready to

☐ be a team player in my health care?

☐ partner with my medical professionals?

☐ be proactive?

☐ invest in my health?

☐ engage with my doctors?

☐ ask questions when I don't understand something?

☐ understand what medications I'm taking?

☐ organize my medical records?

☐ do research on my medical care?

☐ get an advocate when necessary?

3

The Take-Charge Patient's Toolkit
Creating Your Health File, Health Summary, Medical Journal and Medical ID Card

*"Most important is to get copies of your records
at every encounter. Bring copies to your primary
care physician."*

ZOUHDI A. HAJJAJ, MD, INTERNAL MEDICINE,
YARMOUTHPORT, MA

Your Health File

Before you do anything else, start creating your health file. It is the toolkit in which you will create a number of tools to help you be a take-charge patient. Once you have filled your toolkit, you will be off and running. It's just the initial effort that takes a little time.

If you don't create your toolkit, I can promise you there will be a time when you need it and won't have it. Do it now. This could be one of the most important tasks you do as a take-charge patient.

Your health file contains everything that has happened to you medically. It is vital to your medical care because at any time you can withdraw some necessary piece of information that will be pertinent to your current medical care. When you need it most, your health file saves you from having to piece together information so that a doctor can provide you with good care.

You will use information from your health file when you see new doctors, get second opinions, switch doctors, change health insurance,

"It slows us down to call all of these places to track down your medical records—it's wasted time we could be spending with patients."

Charles A. Hunter, MD, FACS, General Surgery, Los Angeles, CA

move to a new town, go to a new medical clinic or hospital or have an emergency. Items from your health file will present a picture about your health and medical status for any doctor to see. It saves time when you really need it.

Even if your doctor or medical facility has electronic medical records, you must have back-up hard copies of all your records. Hard drives crash. Data get lost. Medical staff makes mistakes when they input your information into electronic medical records. There are plenty of horror stories about a patient's medical information getting mixed up with other patients' information, or when medical information is lost. Enough said.

"I have a health file, an 8½ by 11 book filled with copies of all my medical records. I have all my current blood work results, CT scans, PET scans, x-rays—everything that's been done to me is in my file. I have my wife, Joyce, to thank for that."

John O. Will, Patient, Horsham, PA

Your Health File Includes:

- **Your health history**
  - **Surgeries, procedures and tests you've had over your lifetime**
  - **Medical conditions and diagnoses over your lifetime.** These include anything significant that could affect you later on.
- **Your family history**
- **Your medical records:** copies of your pertinent medical records over the last five years
- **Your health summaries,** which include your medications, their dosages, over-the-counter medications, herbs and supplements, and allergies to medications
- **Your medical journal**

- **Doctors:** a list of the doctors you see and what conditions you see them for.
- **Your health insurance:** your insurance company policy and contact information

Your Health History

You will create an overview of significant medical events over your lifetime. This is a one-time effort, and it is the biggest tool in your toolkit.

Your health history gives any new medical professional a brief overview of significant medical events that have occurred over your lifetime. You can create a very condensed version from your medical records so any new doctor can review it and understand which medical conditions, treatments, surgeries, procedures and tests you've had.

The purpose of the health history is to save time so you have more of it with your doctor. If everything medically significant is on paper, all your doctor has to do is read it over and ask questions.

Surgeries, Procedures and Tests

List surgeries, tests and procedures you've had over your lifetime, their dates and the medical professional who performed them. If you had, for example, a major accident that required surgery when you were young, it could be important later on. My C-section in 1995 turned out to be significant in 2010 because the muscle in that area had a tear.

Medical Conditions and Diagnoses over Your Lifetime

List significant medical conditions and diagnoses you've been given by physicians and other medical professionals. These include anything significant that could affect you later on.

Your Family History

Another tool for your toolkit is your family history. Many new doctors will ask for a short version of your family history, meaning they want to know what kinds of diseases and medical conditions run in your family. When you are in the doctor's office, you may not remember everything. Write a short paragraph ahead of time.

Sample Health History

Mary Smith

Address: 555 South Hill Street, Los Angeles, CA

Phone numbers: Work: 310-555-5555; home: 310-555-0000; cell: 310-555-0055

Primary Care Physician: Martin Smith, MD, 310-222-2222

Spouse: J. Smith. Emergency contact information: cell phone: 310-555-5500

Diagnoses:
- January, 2005: Heart murmur. Dr. Tom Olson, cardiologist, Los Angeles, CA
- December, 2000: Acid reflux. Martin Smith, MD. Prescribed Prevacid for several weeks. Acid reflux stopped.
- 1995: Hypothyroid. Dr. Bernstein, internist, Los Angeles. He prescribed 150 mcg of Synthroid. I am currently on that dose of Synthroid.

Surgeries:
- 1992: Shoulder surgery on right shoulder. Stewart Masterson, MD, orthopedist. No complications. My shoulder is fine now.

Tests:
- Colonoscopies 2000, 2005, 2010. Tom Gray, MD, Los Angeles, CA. One or two polyps found in the first colonoscopy (benign) but none found since.

I have copies of my medical records for the past five years. Please let me know if I should provide them.

What did your parents die of? Which diseases, such as cancer, did your parents, aunts, uncles and siblings have? Did your father have a heart attack at age fifty-five? Your doctor will want to know that.

Your family medical history is very important because genes carry markers for diseases. This only means that you can be predisposed to a disease if a close family member had it. This is simply arming your doctor with information in case something comes up.

Example of a condensed family history:

- Father, living, age 68, mild hypertension well controlled by medication.
- Mother, deceased age 65, liver cancer.
- Maternal grandmother, deceased age 86, breast cancer.
- Brother, living, age 35, healthy.

Your Medical Records

Obtain your medical records from each doctor you've seen over the last five years.

- Call each doctor you've seen over the last five years and ask to speak to the medical records department or the front office staff. Ask for copies of your pertinent medical records from the last five years. Explain to this person that you are putting together your own health file for personal use. This will include
  - o test results;
  - o reports from procedures and surgeries;
  - o copies of MRIs and scans.
- You may have to write a letter and fax it to the doctor's office to get copies of your records, and you may have to pay a small fee.
- Communicate with your doctor about why you are asking for copies of your medical records. Some may be afraid that you are moving on to a new doctor or are preparing for a lawsuit. Simply say, "I am putting together my own personal health file. I am very satisfied with your care and will remain your patient. I'm simply trying to get more involved in my health care."
- Sometimes obtaining copies of your medical records can be delayed, so when you make the request, write down the date and to whom you spoke.

Keep in mind that you will not be lugging five years of medical records to a new doctor. If she asks for information, you will have it in your file

> "I have patients who get a copy of their labs or x-rays every time and keep a concurrent file on themselves."
>
> Jack C. Rosenfeld, MD,
> Family Medicine and Geriatrics,
> Lansdale, PA

and you can make copies of what she needs and take them to her.

Place your medical records in your health file. There may come a time when a doctor will ask to see a copy of an MRI you had done. Instead of calling the imaging center or the doctor who ordered it, you will have it in your health file.

From now on, each time you see a doctor and any kind of test is done, ask for a copy of the medical record from that visit. Place it in your health file. This includes test results such as blood work, x-rays, MRIs, CT scans, etc.

Under the HIPAA (Health Insurance Portability and Accountability Act) doctors are legally required to give patients the information they ask for in the format they ask for. For more information on this go to http://www.hhs.gov/ocr/privacy/.

If You Have Problems Obtaining Your Medical Records, Follow These Steps:

- If you have sent in a written request and paid a fee to obtain copies of your medical records and you have not received them within two weeks, call your doctor's office and ask to speak to the person in charge of medical records.

- Write down that person's name. Note the time and date you spoke to her or when you left a message on the voicemail.

- Lab results have to come through your doctor. However, these medical records are legally yours. Ask your doctor to send copies to you.

- If you have further trouble getting your medical records from your doctor's office, send a certified letter to your doctor letting her know that you requested your medical records on (date) and spoke to (name) and paid the fee. Explain that you would like her help. If you still do not hear back from the doctor or the office staff, call the doctor.

- If all else fails, call your local medical association or state medical board and file a complaint with the U.S. Department of Health and Human Service's Office of Civil Rights.

"I was rear ended in a car accident while on vacation in Montana. It resulted in a rib fracture, other bruised ribs, and a concussion. I brought my chest x-ray from Montana to my orthopedist in a suburb of PA. He ordered a bone scan which was done at a local hospital. I brought the bone scan report and the medical record from the orthopedist to my HMO internist. I brought a copy of the orthopedist's notes, bone scan report, plus the orthopedist's and internist's exam notes as well as lab studies to the neurologist in Philadelphia. All three doctors were part of three different health networks. By bringing the records with me, it made it much easier for them to treat me and each knew what the other had done, was doing, was thinking about, and was planning to do."

Joseph J. Morgan, MD, Yardley, PA

Your Health Summary

Another important tool in your health file is your health summary. You create a health summary before each medical encounter. It differs from your health history in that it is an up-to-date account of what has happened physically since you last saw a particular doctor. You may choose to bring a health summary rather than a health history when you see a new doctor, depending on whom you are seeing and why. Keep your old health summaries in your health file.

It is a very brief document that lists your top three medical concerns, a brief description about how you have been feeling, your symptoms, any recent tests, procedures or surgeries you've had, any new medications you are taking and medications you've tried and stopped. It is also a good place to list any questions you have.

Your health summary is your most current health profile. Keep it to about one-half page in length. You are presenting a brief summary in an organized fashion that will keep you and your doctor on track and remind you both of important issues.

Whether I see a new doctor or a doctor I already have a relationship with, I always create a health summary and include copies of recent test or procedure results that pertain to that visit. During my chronic medical condition, I created a health summary for each doctor. I did exactly what I am asking you to do.

Most doctors read my health summaries and every single one was placed into my chart. This was helpful for future visits with my doctors. A big benefit was that those health summaries kept me and the doctors on track and kept my case from appearing confusing and disorganized.

The reason you are being asked to do this kind of preparation is so the doctor doesn't have to waste time digging for information on you. If you have your health summary, complete with your current medical issues or primary complaints, your doctor doesn't have to spend time trying to piece together a full picture of you. You are supporting your doctor's efforts, not replacing them.

Information about You
Include your name, address, date of birth, and emergency contact information.

Contact Information for Other Doctors You Are Currently Seeing
Include their names, phone numbers, and what they are treating you for.

Insurance Information
Include the name of your insurance company.

Primary Complaints
As part of your health summary, create create a list of your top three medical concerns in order of importance along with symptoms you're experiencing.

"Patients don't always think their symptoms are important, relevant or significant. Let the doctor be the judge."

Rae, Registered Nurse, Beverly Hills, CA

Keep track of your symptoms in a medical journal. (See "Create Your Medical Journal" later in this chapter.) Any notebook or pad of paper will do. Your medical journal will provide necessary information for your health summary.

Some patients don't want to complain. Keeping your symptoms to yourself will not help your doctor help you. That is what she is there for—to listen to you and to learn what is happening with you physically. Resist the temptation to minimize your symptoms. If your pain is a nine on a scale of one to ten, it is a nine and your doctor needs to know.

If you have seen another doctor for a medical issue prior to the appointment with the doctor you are currently visiting, be sure to write that down and bring a copy of the medical record with you from that visit. Not all doctors send reports to one another. If you bring your own copy, this saves time so you have more of it with your doctor.

You may have seen another doctor who put you on new medications or asked that you have tests or procedures—this is important to tell your doctor. Physicians are not wizards and today many do not have the time to keep up with other doctors who have seen their patients. It is your job to fill them in. You can help your doctor see the entire picture.

> *"One of my patients had a bleeding ulcer. She was an elderly woman, seventy-four years old. I kept her off of aspirin. Ten years later, she saw a cardiologist who put her back on aspirin. She started to bleed again. She told me that the cardiologist told her to take it and that she had forgotten to tell him about her ulcer. Even if she hadn't remembered, she could have had a file that the doctor could have read. Patients assume doctors look over your charts before you come. You have to remind them."*
>
> Linda Nadwodny, DO, FAAFP, Family Medicine, Lansdale, PA

Diagnoses

If you have been given a diagnosis by the doctor you are visiting or by another doctor, include it in your health summary.

Recent Tests and Procedures

If you have had a test, procedure or surgery since you last saw this physician, list it, along with where it was performed, the date, the doctor and the results. Include copies of test and other results if you feel they are necessary.

Also include copies of other recent test results, MRIs and scans that pertain to your current medical issues and what you've been treated for.

Current Medications and Medication Allergies

> *"I had a new patient who was older. She comes in and says, 'I'm having pain in my legs.'" I find out her blood pressure was out of control. I asked her if she's been diagnosed with high blood pressure before and she said yes, but didn't remember the name of the medication that was prescribed. She had her son with her and he didn't know. I tried to get a list of past surgeries, list of*

medical diagnoses. She was very vague. It was almost a wasted visit because she knew nothing about her medical condition, didn't know the names of medications she was taking. We had to reschedule the visit. I asked her to bring in all the pill bottles for our next visit."

Darlene Petersen, MD, Family Medicine, Roy, UT

Your health summary also includes your list of current medications, over-the-counter medications, herbs and supplements. Hormones are a medication. St. John's wort is a medication, even if it doesn't require a prescription. Herbs and supplements are medications too! I cannot tell you how many doctors said to me, "Patients don't think aspirin is a medicine because it is purchased over the counter. They don't think their vitamins, herbs or supplements count." They count!

"Patients come in and I give them a medication. The next time I see them, I ask how that medication is going. They say, 'I'm not taking it.' They never told me. If you experience side effects you can't tolerate, call the doctor, explain what is happening and ask if you can try something else. Work with the doctor."

Darlene Petersen, MD,
Family Medicine, Roy, UT

List the dosages for each medication and how often you take it. List the brand and generic names—this is for your benefit in case you see another doctor who wants to prescribe a medication you might already be taking. You can check your health summary to make sure she isn't giving you the generic form of a brand medication you are already taking. Many patients get confused with brand and generic names of medications, myself included. Your medications might have changed since you last saw your doctor. Be smart. List everything, even eye drops. List any allergies to medications.

You may think all of this information is in your chart at the doctor's office. It might be, but it may not be up to date. Medications change. Charts get misplaced. Incorrect information about you can be entered into your chart.

Even if your doctor's office has electronic records, it doesn't mean that your records are updated regularly. There can be mistakes with electronic records too. With everything you've learned so far, you'll remember that

Sample Health Summary

Jane Smith

DOB: 5/26/1975

Home Phone: 800-555-1000

Cell Phone: 800-555-1100

Primary Care Physician: Todd Raskin, MD, Internist, Los Angeles, CA
(800-555-1212)

Blue Cross: PPO

Primary Complaints: Stomach pain, burning in throat, belching.
Symptoms are worse after eating, and at night when I lie down.
Maalox and Pepto-Bismol have helped a little. I stopped drinking
diet sodas and eating acidic foods but symptoms still persist.

Current Medications: Flexeril 5mg as needed for muscle pain, Advil
every day for lower back pain, Ambien 10mg as needed.

New Medication: Motrin 100 mg 3x a day.

Questions: What should I do for these symptoms? Is there a
medication I can try? Are there foods I should stay away from to
help alleviate the symptoms? What is this caused by? Do I need
to see a specialist?

doctors and their staff are pressed for time and things can slip through the
cracks. You can support their efforts and doing so will benefit you.

If you have a problem with a medication, write it down in your health
summary. If the doctor prescribed a medication you cannot tolerate, write
down the side effects and what the problem was. You also must call your
doctor about it when this occurs. Tell her how the new medication has
made you feel. This way, she can offer you alternatives.

Many doctors told me that patients don't let them know when a
medication isn't working for them. There are alternatives to medications
that have intolerable side effects. Unless you let your doctor know, she
cannot offer you any other options.

Create Your Medical Journal

As a take-charge patient, you are in collaboration with your doctor. Keeping track of your medical concerns and issues supports you as a team player with your doctor. It also gives you confidence.

Create a medical journal for yourself so you can make notes at the time you think of things. Your medical journal can include

- notes to yourself, reminders;

- lists of questions for your doctor;

- a list of symptoms and when they occur;

- a list of your top concerns;

- notes on conversations you've had with doctors or other medical professionals, suggestions they've made for treatment plans, new medications they have prescribed and more;

- notes on research you may have done on your diagnosis and treatment plan.

If you are currently experiencing symptoms, carry your medical journal with you or take notes in it when you get home. As symptoms occur, write down what they are, where they are located on your body, what time of day they occur, and any events that are associated with the symptoms. For example, you ate lunch and developed stomach pain. What did you eat? Also note what makes symptoms better or worse. For example, if exercise or eating affects your symptoms, write it down. Take your medical journal to every single visit with a medical professional.

No one can remember all the details of a conversation with a physician. You may be nervous. You're in an uncomfortable environment that is unfamiliar. You may be worried about a medical condition or you may not feel well. All of these can interfere with your memory. Taking notes not only allows you to refer to the information later, but it

> "A patient's memory and ability to recall information is profoundly affected by their anxiety and the amount of new information they are exposed to."
>
> David A. Rapkin, PhD, Clinical and Health Psychologist, Mind-Body Medicine Group, Division of Head and Neck Surgery, UCLA David Geffen School of Medicine, Los Angeles, CA

also affords you the freedom to share the information with your loved ones. Conversations with loved ones can often clarify what you have just heard.

I don't know what I would have done without my medical journal during my chronic medical condition. Particularly if you have no accurate diagnosis, you must keep a list of symptoms. I did. I have a small notebook filled with dates, times, what symptoms occurred and when they got worse or better. I was able to use the information in my medical journal when I conversed with my physicians about my medical condition and the pain that accompanied it. The information I provided from my medical journal offered my doctors more information than if I had tried to remember it all. I was also able to refer to the information later.

Create Your Medical ID Card

Your medical ID card is one of the most important tools in your toolkit. As a take-charge patient, you must create a medical ID card. This is something you will carry in your wallet. It doesn't have to be anything fancy or professional. It can be a piece of paper the size of your driver's license or state ID card. I have mine printed on a sheet of paper, folded and slipped into one of the card slots in my wallet next to my driver's license.

If you are traveling or have an emergency, you may not have your health file with you. If you think that one of those computerized chips that goes on your keychain is going to suffice, think again. The EMT who picks you up in an ambulance to take you to the hospital may not have a computer to plug your flash drive into. Besides, computers crash. Electricity shuts down. Data get lost. It's best to keep a hard copy of basic information in your wallet.

You can make a copy of the sample on the next page. You can laminate it but that could make it difficult to keep things up to date.

Your Medical ID Card Should Contain the Following Information:

- Your full name.
- Your primary care physician's name and contact information or the name of any other medical professional who manages your care. This is the person you see the most for your primary care.

```
┌ ─ ─ ─ ─ ─ ─ ─ ─ ─ ─ ─ ─ ─ ─ ─ ─ ─ ─ ─ ─ ─ ─ ─ ─ ─ ─ ─ ─ ─ ┐
│              MEDICAL ID CARD                                │
│ Patient Name: _____     │
│ Home Address: _____     │
│ PCP: _____     │
│ Other Specialists Currently Seeing:                         │
│ _____     │
│ _____     │
│ Current Medications: _____     │
│ Allergies to Medications: _____     │
│ Current Medical Conditions: _____     │
│ Current Diagnoses:_____     │
├ ─ ─ ─ ─ ─ ─ ─ ─ ─ ─ ─ ─ ─ ─ ─ ─ ─ ─ ─ ─ ─ ─ ─ ─ ─ ─ ─ ─ ─ ┤
│                                                             │
│ Emergency Contacts: _____     │
│ Spouse or Partner: _____     │
│ _____     │
│ Friend or Family Member:                                    │
│ _____     │
│ Caregiver if Applicable:                                    │
│ _____     │
│ Preferred Hospital: _____     │
│ Health Insurance: _____     │
│ _____     │
└ ─ ─ ─ ─ ─ ─ ─ ─ ─ ─ ─ ─ ─ ─ ─ ─ ─ ─ ─ ─ ─ ─ ─ ─ ─ ─ ─ ─ ─ ┘
```

- Your current medical conditions, medications and their dosages, over-the-counter medications, including herbs and supplements, and allergies to medications.

- Emergency contact names and phone numbers. List the person you want to be called if you have a medical emergency.

Health Insurance Information

Health insurance is a subject most of us detest. I detest it too but I've had to deal with a lot of it lately and frankly, I wish I'd been more informed before I got ill. I found out the hard way that certain doctors, surgery centers, pathology labs and anesthesiologists weren't covered by my insurance plan.

Now, every time I see a doctor or other medical professional, or schedule a procedure at a hospital or surgery center, I ask ahead of time, "Is this covered by my health insurance?"

Your health insurance is an important part of your toolkit. Place a copy of your health insurance information in your health file. Keep copies of your "Explanation of Benefits" (EOBs) either in your health file or in a separate health insurance file. All the information you receive about health insurance coverage must be kept.

If you don't understand your health insurance coverage, ask someone who does to explain it to you or call the customer service number on the back of your health insurance card.

If you don't know what your insurance plan covers, get to know it now. Better now than when you need it the most—in an emergency.

Please see Chapter 15 on health insurance for more information.

The Medical Information Bureau

This is a reporting agency for the health industry and it may have a file on you. It provides background information to insurance companies to help them determine whom they will provide insurance to.

If you have any errors in your medical records, correct them now. You don't want mistakes landing in this agency's records.

Medical Information Bureau: http://www.mib.com

Correct Errors in Your Medical Records

Once you have received your medical records, review them for accuracy. You might be surprised to find errors in your records.

A word of caution—never let a medical error in your chart go unchallenged. Your medical history follows you for your lifetime. If your doctor takes health insurance and a claim is submitted with an incorrect diagnosis, this could cause your health insurance company to assume that you have a preexisting condition you never had. Better to catch it before you get to that point because if you are ever in need of medical treatment and can't get it because of a medical error made by your doctor's staff, you won't want to hassle with it then. Be prepared and proactive. If there is an error, ask for it to be corrected now.

By law you have the right to correct most errors you find in your medical records. These corrections are called amendments.

Which Medical Records to Review for Errors

- Your doctors' and other medical professionals' records about your visit
- Medical test results
- Medical records from hospitals or other facilities where you have been a patient
- Insurance billing and codes

If you don't understand your medical records, simply call your doctor's office and ask to speak to a nurse. Ask her to explain them to you. You can even make an appointment with that nurse and ask her to go over them with you.

How to Correct Errors in Your Medical Records

Any type of information that will have an effect on your diagnosis, treatment or the ability to get health insurance in the future should be corrected immediately.

- You can call the doctor's office that made the error and ask to speak to the doctor about it.
- If you cannot reach the doctor, ask the front desk person or the nurse for a form they require for making amendments to your medical records.
- Make a copy of the page with the medical error. Either meet with your doctor or fax it to her. Strike a line through the error and ask your doctor to sign it.
- If you need to contact your health insurance company, write a letter, state the date you saw the doctor, copy the page with the medical error with the line through it, and write the correction as it should read. Ask your doctor to sign it.
- Make a copy of the letter and amendment form. Mail, fax or deliver your amendment form. Your provider or facility must act upon your

request within sixty days. If they refuse your request, they must contact you in writing.

Why Do I Have to Do All This Work?

All of these suggestions are for your benefit, because you want the best medical care possible. The way you get it, in part, is to take on some responsibility and get organized, even if it means some work. I won't kid you—some of this is boring but it gets a lot easier once the initial job is done.

Your doctor has something you want that you cannot give to yourself. Make the most of it and do your part by being a take-charge patient. The rest is easy.

PATIENT CHECKLIST

☐ Have I prepared my health file?

☐ Health File includes:
  - Your health history
    - Surgeries, procedures and tests you've had over your lifetime
    - Medical conditions and diagnoses over your lifetime
  - Your family history
  - Your medical records
  - Your health summaries, which include your medications, their dosages, over-the-counter medications, herbs and supplements, and allergies to medications
  - Your medical journal
  - Doctors: a list of the doctors you see and what conditions you see them for.
  - Your health insurance: your insurance company policy and contact information

☐ Have I started my medical journal?

☐ Have I created my medical ID card?

4

How to Choose the Best Doctor for You

"Find a doctor you can trust on a gut level.
Because if you don't trust your doctor, you won't take
their advice."

DAVID BARON, MD, FAMILY MEDICINE, MALIBU, CA,
FORMER CHIEF OF STAFF,
SANTA MONICA-UCLA MEDICAL CENTER & ORTHOPAEDIC HOSPITAL

As take-charge patients, we all need primary care physicians (PCP). Primary care physicians can be internists, family physicians, general practitioners and more. Having a PCP is extremely important, as we all need a "captain of the ship," so to speak, someone who can look at the whole picture even if we see specialists.

Finding a primary care physician with whom you can have a long-term relationship is key to getting good medical care. Some specialists, such as gynecologists and cardiologists, also act as primary care physicians. The same rules apply.

Your relationship with your primary care physician may be one of the most important relationships in your life. Choose a PCP whose personality you like because you may end up spending years with this doctor. The quality of the relationship between you and your doctor defines the quality of care. Most doctors agreed with this.

> "If you don't feel comfortable right from the start, that discomfort will continue. The doctor-patient relationship is one of the most intimate relationships in your life."
>
> Dominic D. Patawaran, MD,
> Family Medicine,
> Los Angeles, CA

Finding a physician who you work well with is very important. You need to feel comfortable with your doctors, no matter how uncomfortable the experience is. Don't undervalue your gut-level impressions. If you meet a provider you are not comfortable with or are not comfortable in her medical facility, pay attention! This gut feeling should factor into your decision about whether you want to see this doctor or not.

Keep in mind that when you find a new primary care physician or a specialist who also acts as a primary care physician, you are actually taking on a relationship not only with the doctor but also with the doctor's practice. You may see a nurse practitioner, a physician's assistant or another doctor in the practice if your doctor is not available. When you meet the doctor, ask about the other medical professionals in her practice.

How to Find a Good Doctor

> "Start with one good physician and she can refer you to other good physicians. Good physicians will know other good physicians like themselves."
>
> Robert J. Adair, MD, FACS,
> Ear Nose and Throat,
> Santa Monica, CA

Finding the best doctor for you is essential for getting the best medical care. You may have a lifelong relationship with your primary care doctor so you want to find the best match for you right from the start. Listed below are several strategies for finding a good doctor and for choosing one who best serves your needs. It's too easy to fall into a relationship with a doctor you aren't really fond of or don't feel as much confidence in as you would like. Take the time now to find a physician who is a good fit, has a good reputation, and whom you trust. You may not have that option when you are in serious need.

- Get a referral from a doctor you already think is very good.

- Get a referral from a friend, relative or colleague you trust. You'll end up hearing names over and over. Pick those that come up more than once.

- If you have a specialist you respect, ask who she sees or recommends to patients. Ask her office staff, such as the nurse, which doctors she sees and likes.

- You can also ask pharmacists for referrals to doctors.

- One doctor suggested asking the charge nurse at a large metropolitan hospital. Other doctors suggested talking to an RN in the emergency room of a local hospital. They said that these nurses know which doctors respond quickly to pages, which doctors visit patients in the hospital and which ones are conscientious.

Research a Doctor's Credentials

Once you compile a list of doctors and their contact information, you'll begin a little research.

It might be tempting to simply rely on referrals for doctors, but it's better to make the time to research a doctor because you can uncover information that others may not know or may not want to tell you.

What to Do:

You'll start by looking up a doctor on the internet simply by name, MD after her name, and the city she is located in.

- What are her credentials? Is she an MD, DO, or something else? What is her specialty? For example, is she an internist with a subspecialty in endocrinology? If you have a certain medical condition, try to find a doctor who has that specialty. For example, if you have a thyroid problem or diabetes, seek out a PCP with endocrinology as a specialty, or find a board-certified endocrinologist who is also a PCP.

"A patient must be extremely careful and selective when getting referred to a doctor or specialist. If the referral is to a doctor in a university setting, the doctor is continually reviewed by his/her peers. If the doctor is in private practice, it is hard to know if he/she is a good doctor."

Lawrence S. Miller, MD,
Clinical Professor,
UCLA David Geffen School
of Medicine, Los Angeles, CA

- You want to find a doctor who is board certified in her specialty. "Certified" means that the doctor has completed a training program in a specialty and has passed an exam to assess her knowledge, skills and experience to provide quality patient care in that specialty. Primary care doctors also may be certified as specialists.

  It is, however, possible to receive good quality care from doctors who are not board certified. You might be surprised to know that many doctors are not board certified.

- Call the office of the doctor you are interested in. Ask the front desk person to give you that doctor's CV. This will list the doctor's credentials, board certification, specialty and which hospitals she is affiliated with. You can pick it up or have it emailed, mailed or faxed to you.

- Pay attention to which hospitals this doctor is affiliated with. A major medical institution is nice, but not always necessary. Any doctor you choose should be affiliated with the hospital of your choice.

- Call the American Medical Association (AMA) for information on training, specialties and board certification of many licensed doctors in the United States. This information also can be found on the AMA website by clicking the "Patients" tab and then "DoctorFinder."

Patient Evaluations of Doctors on the Internet

You can go to websites such as Ratemds.com, Findadoc.com, Vitals.com and more. These sites consist of patients' personal opinions of doctors. These websites have some value, however, you don't know the people who post their opinions. They may have had grievances with a doctor or her office that have nothing to do with the care provided.

I'm not advocating for these websites, but sometimes they come in handy.

Trust Your Instincts

You have to have confidence and trust in your doctor. This may take a couple of visits to develop, but in that first visit, trust your instincts. Find a doctor you have a good rapport with. If you believe your doctor has your best interests at heart and understands you, you'll be more willing to follow her advice.

As I mentioned earlier, the urogynecologist I saw almost a year into my chronic pelvic pain condition put me at ease right away and I immediately felt confidence in her ability to help me. I'd seen many doctors before her who appeared as confident as she did, but almost none exhibited a sound belief that they were going to help me get better. To make my decision even easier, she has an excellent reputation, is board certified in her specialty and is affiliated with a highly respected medical school.

Find a Doctor Who Welcomes Your Participation in Your Care

As a take-charge patient, you'll want to find a doctor who welcomes your questions, is willing to go over your concerns and is open to discussing research on your specific medical issue, medication or treatment plan. A good doctor wants you to fully understand what she is proposing and is willing to discuss it, even if briefly, so you are on board with her diagnosis and treatment plan.

> "Medicine has created a very paternalistic relationship between doctors and their patients. It's easier to practice medicine that way. You do what I tell you and that's it. But ultimately, it's not in the patient's best interest. The passive approach on the part of the patient, does not work."
> Linda Nadwodny, DO, FAAFP, Family Medicine, Lansdale, PA

You Have to Feel Heard and Understood

Keep in mind that while on your search for a doctor, whomever you meet with must take time with you. You must feel listened to. This means you and the doctor communicate well. Good communication is essential to a successful doctor-patient relationship and that translates to much better medical care. Good communication means that you understand what the doctor is talking about and that the doctor understands you. If you don't understand her medical jargon, it doesn't mean this doctor is out of the running for you. Simply ask questions about the terminology and take responsibility for asking for clarification.

Can the Doctor See You When You Are Ill?

In your decision-making process, think about how important it is for you to have a doctor who will see you when you are sick.

"You can run a practice in a rigid or flexible manner. If you choose a flexible method the physician allots the necessary time for the patient and does not stick to a rigid schedule. That type of practice also tends to add patients with urgent problems to the daily schedule even if it makes them behind in the schedule and results in delays in seeing other patients. You can't have that type of availability and flexibility in time spent with the patient and keep a perfect schedule. You don't always know what a patient has when they come in. They could have a sore throat which will take ten minutes or they have throat cancer and that takes forty-five minutes."

Robert J. Adair, MD, FACS,
Santa Monica, CA

You have to ask questions to find out. In order to strick to their time schedules, some doctors do not make room for same-day appointments. They do not want to make other patients wait. There are pros and cons to each type of doctor.

Doctors generally run their offices in two ways—rigid or flexible.

If you don't want to run late, choose a doctor who runs a rigid practice. If you want to be seen when you are sick, choose a doctor who will fit you in. If you choose the latter, keep in mind that you might have to wait when the doctor fits in other patients who are in need.

Choose a Doctor Who Will Return Your Phone Calls

Finding a doctor who returns your phone calls may not seem important now, but if you are sick or need her help, a return phone call will be important. This does not mean a return phone call in the middle of the day unless it is a true emergency or a return phone call on the weekend if she is not on call. If you leave a message, most doctors will return your call at the end of the day or on the next business day. It happens occasionally that the doctor doesn't get the message that you called or was called away on an emergency. Call again, but be mindful of this if it becomes a pattern.

Above all, you'll want to trust and rely on a doctor and have confidence in her as a professional.

Questions to Think About before You Meet a Doctor

- Do you feel more comfortable with a male or female doctor? With some specialties, this might make a difference to you.

- Do you want a doctor who speaks your language or who is from the same culture? Many medical professionals recommended this because it makes practicing good medicine so much easier. You could get better medical care if you choose a doctor who understands your norms, your culture and your language.

- Do you want a doctor who is close to your home? Within fifteen minutes? Thirty minutes?

- Do you want a doctor who will see you if you are in the hospital? If so, you must ask this question of the doctor's office staff before your visit. Some doctors do not visit their patients in the hospital. Either they have specified doctors in their practice who visit all their patients or a hospitalist sees all the patients there.

  I was very surprised to find out that my specialist did not come to see me when I was in the hospital. Instead I was seen by one of the new doctors in her practice whom I had never met before.

- Do you need a doctor affiliated with the hospital you most likely will go to? You probably do. Before you meet a doctor, ask the front office staff which hospitals she is affiliated with. If you do have to be in a hospital, you will want your doctor to see you there, and if she does not have privileges at your hospital, she will not be able to. Try to have all your doctors affiliated with the same hospital so they can communicate with one another.

- Do you need to see a doctor on weekday evenings or on Saturdays? Ask questions of the doctor's front office staff before you make the appointment.

Questions to Ask the Front Office
Before You Make That First Appointment

"When choosing a physician, one question to ask is if electronic health records (EHR) are used for patient records. If not, run for the hills. It tells you that the physician thinks the investment isn't worth it. Electronic health records are a patient advocate tool and if a physician isn't invested in that, it's telling."

David Lee Scher, MD, FACP, FACC, FHRS, Harrisburg, PA

Simply say to the doctor's front office staff, "I'm looking for a new doctor and I'd like to ask a few questions before I make an appointment."

Here are a few suggestions. You might want to take notes while you are talking to the doctor's front desk person.

- Does the doctor take my health insurance or Medicare, etc.? Ask if the doctor plans on continuing to take your health insurance. There are no guarantees, but ask anyway.
- How many patients does the doctor see in a day?
- How long do patients have to wait in the waiting room before their appointments?
- How long does it usually take to get a routine appointment?
- How long does it take to get a sick appointment?
- Will the doctor fit me in if I really need to see her?
- How much time does the doctor usually spend with a patient?
- If you are into alternative medicine, is the doctor involved in or open to alternative medicine?
- Is the doctor's practice affiliated with an urgent care center?
- Is the office wheelchair accessible?
- Which hospitals is the doctor affiliated with?
- Does the doctor's practice use a website for appointments, education or advice?
- Does the doctor have a nurse practitioner or physician's assistant?

You may not be able to get everything you want in one doctor. Make a list of your top five priorities and start from there. Remember, you might have to meet with more than one doctor to find one you connect with. Just because a close friend likes a doctor doesn't mean that you will. Trust your instincts.

Remember to Evaluate the Doctor's Staff

Since you will be interacting with a doctor's staff on a regular basis, evaluate the office staff as you talk to them on the phone and also as you approach the desk to sign in. Are they polite? Do they greet you? Are they pleasant? Do you feel welcome? Are they rude or dismissive? Look around the waiting room. If a patient is complaining, this could be a red flag. Pay attention.

Keep in mind that over the years when you see this doctor, it will be the doctor's nurse or medical assistant who may be taking your blood pressure and vital signs. Do you feel comfortable and welcomed by these people?

When to Look for Another Doctor

Some of us stick with doctors we don't care for. There is no reason to see a doctor who disrespects you, dismisses you, doesn't listen to you or is condescending in any way. There are too many good doctors to put up with that. If you do, your treatment is likely to be compromised.

If you happen to be with a doctor you aren't crazy about, you might resist looking for a new one because it takes time and it's just so easy to put off. You might think you won't need to see your doctor for a while anyway because you're fit and healthy.

Think again.

You'll regret having a doctor you don't like when you are in need. Imagine not feeling well or being very sick and having to find a new doctor. Do it when you are well and while you can.

Being a take-charge patient is being a prepared patient. Prepare now. Spend a little time and effort to find a doctor you feel comfortable with and like as a person. You have to be able to communicate with a doctor. If you can't, find another one.

Here is a list of possible red flags. If your doctor displays these behaviors frequently, you might want to look for another one.

> "I used to see an excellent specialist who many of my friends saw as well. I went to him for years. His staff was consistently rude to all of us. Everyone I knew stopped seeing him because of the staff. The doctor had always been nice to me and I thought he was an excellent doctor. It was not until he lost his temper with me one day that I figured out that doctors may choose staff who are more like them than we think."
>
> Anonymous Patient, Miami, FL

> "There are doctors who approach being doctors like car salesmen and are focused on making money."
>
> David A. Rapkin, PhD, Clinical and Health Psychologist, Mind-Body Medicine Group, Division of Head and Neck Surgery, UCLA David Geffen School of Medicine, Los Angeles, CA

Your Doctor Takes Phone Calls during Your Office Visit

Does your doctor take phone calls while you are in the exam room with her? A number of patients complained about this, and a few doctors warned about doctors who take calls while they are with you.

I have one doctor who takes calls only when it is important. He spends a lot of time with me so I don't mind. But I would mind if our office visit lasted under fifteen minutes and it took me a month to get in to see him. Keep in mind that this is your time.

Your Doctor Always Makes You Wait

If you see a doctor regularly, and she consistently makes you wait an hour or two, you might consider finding another doctor. If you like your doctor and want to stick with her, talk to her about this and open up a discussion about the amount of time you are regularly forced to wait. Be careful not to put her on the defensive. You can say something like this: "Dr. Smith, I like you as my doctor. You've helped me a lot through the years and I appreciate everything you've done for me. But it's very difficult for me as a working parent to wait as long as I do every time I come to see you. Is there anything we can do about this?"

> "A lot of doctors forget that their patients are also busy."
>
> Dominic D. Patawaran, MD,
> Family Medicine,
> Los Angeles, CA

Some doctors are late for legitimate reasons such as patient emergencies, surgeries that run overtime or because of patients with urgent needs who require more time in an office visit.

However, some doctors make you wait because they can. Some double book patients to try to see as many as they can in a day. There's not much you can do in this case because frankly, you are at their mercy. If you want to see another doctor to avoid delays, then do that. But if you see a doctor who makes you wait and you believe this doctor is the best match for you, allow extra time when you see her. Sometimes it's just the way it is. I don't like it either.

Your Doctor Takes Extended Vacations

Does your doctor take extended vacations? Doctors need time off too but some can take many weeks off during the course of a year. If you have a serious or chronic medical issue, a doctor's absence may affect your care. Consider this carefully.

Your Doctor Has a Bad Bedside Manner

If your doctor's bedside manner makes you uncomfortable, then it will affect your relationship with her, and that in turn will affect your medical care. I don't put up with a bad bedside manner unless I am in the emergency room or in the hospital and unable to appoint another doctor. Neither should you.

The only exception might be with an excellent surgeon. I'd put up with a bad bedside manner if I knew the surgeon was the best for what I had and she had the most experience with the type of surgery I needed. I'd rather see a really good surgeon who isn't terribly personable than the opposite. You will see this doctor probably twice or three times and then you are done.

When I was sick, I saw a specialist I'd never met before for a consultation on my chronic pelvic pain. He was immediately hostile toward me as I entered his office. I had prepared my usual health summary, complete with copies of all of my tests, list of medications, symptoms, doctors I'd seen and more. I'd even dressed in a suit because I wanted respect. At this point, he was the sixth doctor I'd seen and I wanted to put my best foot forward.

I had barely said hello when he reprimanded me for not delivering my medical records before the appointment. His nurse had not asked me to do that when I made the appointment but I should have asked.

Seated across the desk from him, I tried my best to be polite and answer all of his questions while he pored over my medical records. He challenged me by staring me down, as if sizing me up in an openly hostile way. Why? I have no idea. But I do know that I will never go back to him.

If you are talked down to, dismissed or disrespected by a doctor, find another. No doctor should ever talk down to you. You are an equal to that doctor. Bad treatment will affect the relationship between you and will compromise your medical care. Some doctors can be arrogant and downright unpleasant. Walk away.

Your Doctor's Attention Is Elsewhere

Is her attention on your chart or on an electronic device? I've heard stories from patients about doctors who rarely looked at them. Instead, they were focused on charts, on electronic devices or spent much of the office visit dictating notes into a recorder.

One patient's daughter told me that every time she takes her eighty-seven-year-old mother to the doctor, he spends part of the time dictating notes into a recorder and rarely looks her mother in the eye. This doctor is sending a message to the patient that she is not as important as his schedule. This is unacceptable. If you have a doctor like this, find another.

You deserve to be respected and treated well. You are paying money for this office visit. Don't put up with bad treatment.

I want to make one caveat regarding the above information. Doctors are human beings and they have bad days just like you and I do. They may not have slept well the night before, may have been up with a new baby most of the night, may have had some bad news the day before or had an argument with their spouse that morning. If a doctor normally treats you respectfully and with warmth, you might write off a couple of negative interactions to humanness.

PATIENT CHECKLIST

☐ Have I found a primary care physician?

☐ Am I satisfied with my current doctor?

☐ Have I found referrals if I need to find a new doctor?

☐ Have I researched the new doctor's credentials?

☐ Have I called the new doctor's office to ask questions?

☐ Have I evaluated the doctor's staff?

5

Your Relationship with Your Doctor

"A good relationship with your physician can lead to better medical care."

ZOUHDI A. HAJJAJ, MD, INTERNAL MEDICINE,
YARMOUTHPORT, MA

Your relationship with your doctor is an important one that can last for many years. It is a partnership. You and your doctor collaborate to maintain your good health and to treat any medical conditions, illnesses or injuries that occur. A good doctor-patient relationship includes mutual trust, respect and good communication.

Trust

Finding a doctor you trust isn't always easy. If you're given a good recommendation by another doctor or loved one you trust, then it's more likely you'll find what you're looking for. Trust is personal and it is what your relationship with your physician is based on. It takes faith and plenty of reliable experiences with the same person to develop it. It also involves trusting your own instincts.

"Establish a relationship with a doctor who you can trust and have confidence in. Decide with your doctor. Have your spouse, relative, friend with you to participate and augment the communication process. Patients can be frightened or emotional when a doctor is communicating with them. Patients don't always recall details of their conversation with their doctor. The spouse, relative or friend can help them remember."

Daniel Wohlgelernter, MD, Cardiology, Santa Monica, CA

Trusting your doctor affects

- your belief in her ability to provide good medical care;
- your willingness to follow her treatment plans;
- your willingness to follow up with recommended procedures and tests;
- how you feel about the care you are given;
- your willingness to take her diagnosis seriously and discuss your concerns without fear of being dismissed;
- and much more.

You must do your part in cultivating trust with your doctor. This means divulging everything and not keeping secrets, following a treatment plan and talking to your doctor if you cannot do so.

This also means approaching your doctor with confidence. Educate yourself about any diagnosis and treatment plan before you follow through with it.

What Can Enhance Trust in Your Doctor

- Your doctor values your contribution to your medical care.
- Your doctor treats you with respect.
- Your doctor listens to you and addresses your concerns.
- You are honest with your doctor.
- You communicate well with your doctor and she with you. This means that the doctor summarizes correctly what you have told her. You both consistently understand what the other is saying.
- You are comfortable asking her questions.

Trust is earned. You and your doctor have to work together to create it.

Mutual Respect

Mutual respect means that you value your doctor's expertise and have faith in the medical care she offers you. In return, you feel that your doctor values you as the patient and trusts what you report to her about your body. This means neither one is condescending or dismissive in your interactions with one another.

I've heard from several patients who had difficult-to-diagnose diseases or multiple medical issues who were afraid that their doctors thought they were crazy or were hypochondriacs. Every time I hear this, I am incensed. I suspect that some doctors blame their patients when they cannot find the correct diagnosis and treatment plan.

Just because a doctor is unable to correctly diagnose your illness or condition or figure out an effective treatment plan, this does not mean you are crazy. It means that no answer has been found yet.

> "There must be mutual respect between a doctor and patient. If the patient doesn't respect the doctor, it's three strikes against the patient. There has to be honesty between doctor and patient, and they must honor each other."
>
> Albert Kaufman, MD, Neurosurgery, Long Beach, CA

People have asked me if doctors treated me as if I were crazy during my sixteen months of chronic pelvic pain when no accurate diagnosis or treatment plan had been found. Each time I am asked, I say that I did my best to prevent that. I approached each doctor as if I was meeting with a business partner. I was in charge as a patient and I arrived in the doctor's office prepared, organized and knowledgeable about my symptoms. Even if I doubted myself at times, I didn't show it. I knew where my pain was located, what made it worse or better, what eased it and exactly how long I'd had it. If a doctor doubted me, I never knew it.

When recently discussing this book with one of my doctors, he told me that the way I interact with him is key to the success of the collaborative aspect of our relationship. He mentioned patients who are not respectful of his expertise and who come right out and tell him what they believe their diagnosis to be. He explained that this approach puts most doctors on the defensive and challenges their egos.

I know my style works well with most physicians because it conveys respect. I ask questions, such as, "Do you think x could be contributing to my medical problem?" rather than making statements like "X is contributing to my medical problem." I defer to doctors in that way because it allows them to act like the experts they are, and they aren't faced with a patient who thinks she knows it all or knows more than they do. Patients who come across as know-it-alls really bug doctors. Now, you may know a lot, especially about your body, but the way you interact with physicians is very important. Acting deferential and conveying respect, even if you don't feel that way, will get you more of what you want.

Communication

Communication is one of the major components of a good relationship with your doctor. If you and your doctor don't communicate well this increases the probability for medical errors, erodes trust, and can ultimately compromise your medical care.

"Communication with the doctor is fundamental to the doctor/patient relationship. Find a doctor and learn early if he/she is a good communicator and will spend the time with you. Find a doctor who will allow patient input and questions. Establish a relationship and make sure you have confidence in the doctor."

Daniel Wohlgelernter, MD,
Cardiology, Santa Monica, CA

Good communication means that you and your doctor work as a team.

Good communication includes

- listening to your doctor;
- feeling listened to and understood;
- focusing on specifics and not veering from your main concerns;
- looking at one another in the eye;
- mutual respect;
- conversing with your doctor, engaging in a dialogue;
- being honest;
- speaking the same language;
- asking questions;
- and more.

How to Address Your Doctor

Several doctors talked about how patients address them and how some use their first names. If you address your doctor by her first name without this informality being established, it can be seen as a challenge. The correct way to address your doctor is by using Dr. and her last name. If you want the best medical care possible, why challenge the doctor's ego, even in a minor way, by using her first name when you meet her?

Speak in an Even Tone

Try not to get overly emotional. Doctors are cognitive thinkers and many have said that it's easier for them to communicate with patients who are not overly emotional, who stay on track, keep things simple and organized and stay on point. Doctors are affected by your demeanor and if you are melodramatic, it can turn your doctor off. You don't want your doctor to stop listening to you.

If you can use medical terminology, you might find that your doctor listens to you more.

Be Honest with Your Doctor

Resist lying or holding things back. Your doctor cannot do her job if you aren't forthcoming. Share your symptoms, bad habits, side effects of medication and medications you have stopped taking and more. If she has recommended a test that you didn't follow though on, tell her. Be upfront.

> "If a patient is afraid to tell me they haven't been taking their meds, it can be dangerous."
>
> Dominic D. Patawaran, MD,
> Family Medicine,
> Los Angeles, CA

Gee, Doc, I'm Scared

If there is something about your health that is scaring you, bring it up to the doctor. It's not easy being vulnerable in this way but keeping it to yourself makes it worse! If you're scared, tell the doctor. You might just get some reassurance that you are not dying of a brain tumor.

For example, "Doctor, I've been worried I might have cancer. My sister was just diagnosed with breast cancer and I have not been feeling well." Then list your symptoms, explain why you are afraid and enter into a conversation about your health.

I'm Embarrassed

Many doctors speculated that patients wait too long to come in for an office visit to discuss symptoms they've been experiencing because they are embarrassed.

This is pretty understandable and I've felt that way myself but waiting until your symptoms have progressed doesn't help you. We all know that, of course, even though some things are really hard to talk about.

If you're embarrassed about a medical condition or about symptoms you're having, know that many of us feel that way. Pick a doctor you feel safe with and get in for an office visit to discuss the problem. If you choose the doctor you are most comfortable with, you might find that it's easier to pick up the phone to make that appointment.

I'm Worried about Cost

If you have financial concerns that affect the medical treatment your doctor prescribes for you, talk to her about it. There are usually less expensive alternatives. Many doctors have good options available to assist patients who are burdened by medical costs.

Communication is essential. Your doctor can't do her job unless you provide the information she needs. It is your responsibility to speak up about any financial issues that might interfere with following through on the medical treatment your doctor recommends for you.

Ask Questions

Full understanding of what a doctor tells you is key to good communication. This includes asking questions if you are confused.

> "Most of us in the medical field do not realize how difficult it is for the average person to understand what a medical professional is saying to them."
>
> Jessica G. Schairer, PhD,
> Clinical and Health
> Psychologist, Los Angeles, CA

Doctors can speak in complicated medical jargon. If you don't understand what she is saying, ask her to explain it in a different way. You can say something like this, "I don't understand why you want me to take this medication or undergo this treatment. Would you please go over it again?"

Be assertive and speak up. If you ask questions, most doctors will respect you for being invested in your care.

If you don't understand why your doctor wants you to take a medication or have a test or procedure, ask for clarification.

Full understanding will ultimately help you commit to your doctor's recommendations. This is part of getting the best medical care.

I Don't Want to Bother the Doctor

Some people are worried about bothering the doctor with questions or concerns. This is understandable because doctors are so busy, but try to keep in mind that this is what they are there for—to serve you. They can't do that unless you tell them what is going on with you.

You must be courageous and speak up, ask questions, be honest about your symptoms and suppress the fear of burdening the doctor. I am intimidated by certain doctors too. What I have learned from my own experience and from interviews with doctors and health psychologists is to approach the doctor in a level-headed and confident fashion.

Doctors are taught in medical school to relay information to patients with confidence. You can use the same method. How I handle it is by adopting a logical and confident manner. I act as if I do not doubt myself even though in some cases I wonder if I am reporting my symptoms or experiences correctly. I act as if I know what I'm talking about when I report what is happening with my body.

I walk into the doctor's office with my health file in hand. I appear as if I am in control, even if I don't feel it. That is why I dress nicely to meet doctors I'm intimidated by. I approach the visit as if I would a business meeting. This increases my confidence.

If all else fails, remember that you are paying your doctor to help you. Think about the bill you are going to receive at the end of the visit and muster the confidence to speak up.

Find a Doctor Who Speaks Your Language

Communication is essential for good medical care. If you do not speak the same language as your doctor and no one on her staff speaks your language, you can always bring in a family member to translate for you. However, many doctors said that family members are not translators and can misinterpret what the doctor is saying.

Stick to the Point

If you speak only about your top three most important medical concerns, it keeps you and your doctor on task. If you stray from the point with details from your personal life that do not pertain to your visit, you'll be wasting your valuable time with the doctor. If you veer off into what your friends and family members told you to do, you will lose the focus and attention of the doctor.

However, it is important to let your doctor know if something important is affecting you—for example, if your parent or spouse just died and you're having trouble dealing with the loss. Your doctor will want to factor that into the overall picture.

Even Take-Charge Patients Need to Listen

Even if you consider yourself to be a medically savvy, take-charge patient, several doctors suggested that you stay open to what they have to say about your medical condition, diagnosis and treatment options. In the end it is up to you to decide whether to act on the advice you are given, but you owe it to yourself and to the physician to take in her opinion and mull it over. Allow the doctor to educate you even if you decide against what she has to offer. In the end, the choice is yours.

> "Let your doctor get a foot in the door. Allow him to educate you even if you decide not to do it. Don't reject his advice immediately. You still have a choice. Listen to what he has to say. You can always ask, 'Do we have any alternatives to that?'"
>
> David Baron, MD, Family Medicine, Malibu, CA, Former Chief of Staff, Santa Monica-UCLA Medical Center & Orthopaedic Hospital

A week after my mother died in 2001, my back went into spasm. I could barely move. I saw an orthopedist. After looking at my MRI, he immediately told me that I needed back surgery to correct two herniated discs. I listened to what this doctor had to say. I asked questions about his reasons for thinking I needed surgery and what surgery might do for me.

I also listened to my gut feeling, which was that I didn't want or need back surgery. My mother had three of them and she ended up in a wheelchair. As I listened to what this doctor said, I paid attention to what I was feeling. My gut instinct was to get a second opinion.

I went for a second opinion with a respected back surgeon who was affiliated with a major medical institution. He looked at my MRI, took x-rays, gave me an exam and said emphatically that I did not need back surgery. He explained that my herniated discs and degenerative disc disease were not debilitating and that I could live comfortably if I exercised enough. He explained that I could expect about one back episode a year.

I did what the surgeon told me to do and acted on his direction because it made sense to me. I live relatively pain free with one or two minor episodes a year.

You Need to Be Listened To

Do you feel that your doctor listens to you? This is a very important aspect of the quality of communication with your doctor. If your doctor is not fully engaged with you, then something needs to change.

> "It's very important for patients to have a doctor who listens to their story. It's a balance for the doctor between time pressure and trying to make money and not rushing through an office visit."
>
> Karlene Ross, MD, Family Medicine, Waldorf, MD

Tips to Maximize the Relationship with Your Doctor

Here are a few suggestions that will help you make the most of your relationship with your doctor. They are for your benefit as a patient, because the more you know, the more empowered you will feel.

Remember That Doctors Are Human Beings

Almost every health care professional emphasized that we all must realize that doctors are people just like us. They have personalities, feelings, good days, bad days, families and social lives.

Sometimes doctors are forced to sacrifice important events to tend to their patients. They miss their kids' soccer games, medical appointments, school meetings and social events. Sure, they chose their profession, but the demands and sacrifices are great. I never realized just how much they sacrifice for their patients until I interviewed the physicians for this book.

> "Doctors are human too. I remember a patient. After seeing me for an office visit, she went back to her primary physician and said, 'I never want to see that doctor again.' The day before I'd seen her, I had just buried my mother."
>
> Alan Jasper, MD, Internal Medicine and Pulmonary Diseases, Los Angeles, CA

Humanize Yourself to Your Doctor

"If you are meeting your doctor for the first time, find common ground. Are they a parent? Through that connection, you get the healthcare provider to see you as a human being, not just as a set of symptoms."

Elizabeth Williams, PhD, Vanderbilt-Ingram Cancer Center, Nashville, TN

It's easy for us to feel the urgency to get right to the point of why we are seeing the doctor. We begin listing symptoms, talk about how we aren't feeling well, and ask for help.

I happen to believe that if we jump right into our symptoms, that is how the doctor will view us—as a set of symptoms she needs to diagnose and treat. I want my doctor to see me as a human being, just as I see her. If she sees me as a human being, then more than likely she will connect to me personally, and that can enhance her willingness to help me. This may not always be possible as some doctors simply are not interested in connecting personally to their patients.

Use Your People Skills

If someone likes you, they are more willing to go the extra mile for you. This is where your people skills are useful because your doctor will respond to you more positively if you are friendly. That isn't always easy if you aren't feeling well, but I've heard from many doctors that a patient who is angry, bitter, belligerent or has a bad attitude is not well liked. Being a likeable patient is being a smart patient.

Being a smart patient doesn't mean you are faking or being disingenuous. It means you implement strategies to maximize your interaction with the doctor and her staff. You don't have to put up with bad treatment or allow anyone to treat you disrespectfully—I'm not suggesting that you be a doormat. I'm suggesting that being a nice person will get you more of what you want.

Be Nice to Your Doctor

Be nice, polite and appreciative. Many doctors shared experiences with me about patients who were not nice to them. If you aren't nice to your doctor, you are not going to get what you want.

Your doctor has something you want that you cannot give to yourself. Do your best to elicit a positive response from your doctor. It's just common sense.

We've all had experiences with doctors who have made us wait forever when we weren't feeling well or whose staff ignored us or were rude or unhelpful. I'm not asking you not to stick up for yourself; I'm asking you to express yourself diplomatically because you need what this doctor has to offer.

I try to show goodwill and appreciation toward my doctors not just from a public relations perspective (although that does factor in), but also because I do truly appreciate what my doctors do for me. I am mindful of how far a simple verbal thank you or thank-you note goes.

The goal is to let your doctor know that you value the good care she gives you. If your doctor goes the extra mile for you, express gratitude. We all like to hear that we have done well or that we have done something to improve someone else's life. Doctors need that too.

If you complain a lot or approach the doctor and staff with a bad attitude or a sense of entitlement, you are simply not going to get what you want. If there has been a serious error or act of obvious neglect, channel your anger so you don't come across as out of control. Remember—be firm but respectful. No name-calling or yelling. You only discredit yourself if you yell at doctors and their staff. You look like the villain if you lose control.

> "A good relationship with the doctor is the cornerstone of keeping the patient healthy."
>
> Damon Raskin, MD, Internal Medicine, Pacific Palisades, CA

> "You need to have a nice relationship with me. When (bleep) hits the fan, you are going to need me."
>
> Jo Ann C. Pullen, MD, Internal Medicine and Geriatrics, Los Angeles, CA

> "Most doctors want to help. They've sacrificed a lot. When they can't, they can feel a sense of personal letdown because they really do identify with people's suffering. Sometimes their training to do everything within their power to cure can backfire, and make them feel a sense of personal failure when they can't."
>
> Roger E. Dafter, PhD, Associate Director, Mind-Body Medicine Group, Division of Head and Neck Surgery, UCLA David Geffen School of Medicine, Los Angeles, CA

Be Nice to the Doctor's Staff

Befriend the doctor's staff. This will help you in a multitude of ways. For example, if you have an urgent message for the doctor, need to see the doctor the same day, need a prescription refill sooner rather than later, or need a procedure scheduled immediately, most of the time you'll get your needs met much sooner if you are friendly and appreciative of the doctor's staff.

Most medical professionals suggested trying to talk with the same person each time you call the office to establish a relationship with that person. This will be your go-to person if you ever have an important need to be addressed.

If the front desk person fits you in for an urgent appointment, thank her. This person did you a favor.

Be Nice to the Doctor on Call

Several doctors mentioned the importance of being polite and respectful to the doctor on call—the physician who is covering for your doctor. If you are not, word gets around. This affects how the doctor and her staff perceive you, and it can affect the quality of your medical care.

Act Involved in Your Health

Who knows your body better than you do? You are the expert on you—share with your doctor what you know so she can do her job.

Most doctors said that patients who are involved and invested in their health cause them to be more involved and invested in the patient's health. Many physicians said that if a patient doesn't care, it makes their job much more difficult. Many said that patients who don't care aren't going to follow their instructions to get better.

If you think about it, what is your doctor's motivation to go out of her way for you if you give the impression you don't care about your health and medical care?

What Can Erode the Doctor-Patient Relationship

You might not have thought about what could erode the relationship between you and your doctor. Think about it now. A good relationship with your medical professional will enhance your care. There are behaviors that will not support what you want—to get the best medical care for you.

The Back-Stabbing Patient

Several doctors I interviewed brought up the patient who complains about previous doctors she has seen. Don't do it. If, in your opinion, the last doctor you saw wasn't good, don't tell the new doctor this. She might view you as a patient who will never be satisfied. This can deflate a doctor's motivation to work with you. This contradicts what you want—to get the best medical care possible.

The Difficult Patient

You can probably guess what a difficult patient is but I'll outline it briefly here, because in the end, if you are difficult it could compromise your care.

Difficult patients

- talk to their doctors as if they know more than the doctors do;
- demand antibiotics or pain medications without being seen by their doctor;
- repeatedly ask to be treated over the phone;
- lie to their doctors;
- are belligerent, rude or nasty;
- are overly demanding.

As take-charge patients, we may think we know what we need medically, and maybe we do at times, but making demands of a doctor will backfire. Be diplomatic as often as you can. Ask questions politely. Respect what the doctor has to say about your medical condition and treatment even if you decide it is not right for you.

You can ask for a test or medication and explain why you think you need it. Accept the doctor's decision if her answer is no. The doctor really is the medical expert, not you. You can bring to the table the knowledge of a take-charge, educated and informed patient, but crossing the line into the category of difficult patient will only disrupt the relationship between you and your doctor.

You can ask your question like this, "My last doctor put me on Lexapro. I did well on that for a long time. Do you think I could try that again?"

Using the Phone

Many doctors reported that their patients call them on the phone for diagnoses and for medications. For minor requests this is acceptable, but if you are sick, think you need an antibiotic or need advice on how you can get better, don't expect your doctor to treat you over the phone. Instead, make an appointment for an office visit. Your doctor needs to see you, make an evaluation and decide what is best for you.

If you need to call your physician, keep in mind that your chart has to be pulled and your request has to go through the front desk or possibly the doctor's nurse. Try to get your questions answered in the office visit with the doctor so you don't have to call back later.

> "I had an older male patient who went to a dermatologist and had a biopsy. It became infected and this patient wasn't able to reach the dermatologist. He called me and demanded a prescription for antibiotics over the phone. He was angry when I told him he'd have to come in for an office visit if he wanted antibiotics. He refused to come in for an office visit. The patient threatened to get another doctor. In the future, I won't go out of my way for a patient like this. I have a strict policy of not giving antibiotics over the phone without a visit. I don't appreciate being told what to do and putting me, as a doctor, at risk."
>
> Bernard P. Ginsberg, MD, Family Medicine, Tavernier, FL

Calling Your Doctor after Hours

Paging the doctor after hours and on weekends is for urgent matters only, not for simple requests that can be handled the next business day. Your doctor has a life too. It is simply not appropriate to page your doctor or call her on her cell phone unless she has given you explicit permission to do so. If you do have an urgent medical situation, have your physician paged and then decide if you need to go to your nearest emergency room.

> "I have a patient who paged me on a weekend morning at 5 AM with the stomach flu. There was nothing I could do for her at that time."
>
> Alison Garb, MD, Internal Medicine, Pacific Palisades, CA

**Alternatives to Calling the Doctor after Hours
with Nonurgent Matters**

- Call your pharmacist. You can discuss over-the-counter remedies to tide you over until the next business day.

- Go to an urgent care center or a retail medical clinic. See Chapter 19 for more information.

- Many health insurance plans have twenty-four hour nurses available for phone consultation. Find out if your insurance provides this.

Tips for Successful Phone Communication

During business hours and during the week, it can be difficult to get in touch with your doctor. She might be in surgery, visiting patients in the hospital or backed up with patients in her office.

- Always give the doctor's office the phone number where you can be reached. There is nothing more frustrating than expecting a phone call from the doctor and missing it. If you give your cell phone number, keep your phone with you and leave it turned on.

- Just as with an office visit, keep your notebook handy and take notes on what the doctor says when she calls.

- Have your pharmacy name and phone number with you in case the doctor wants to call in a prescription.

- Have your current health summary with you so if your doctor asks a question about a medication you are taking, you will have a list of your medications to refer to.

- If you are expecting a phone call from your doctor and you have questions, write them down ahead of time. That way, you are less likely to get caught up in what the doctor is saying and get sidetracked, forgetting important questions you want answered.

Avoid Calling at 4 PM on Friday

Try not to call the doctor's office for answers to questions or for prescription refills late on Friday afternoon. You may not get a return phone call or your prescription refill. Try to plan ahead. This is for your benefit so you can get what you need.

PATIENT CHECKLIST

☐ Do I trust my doctor?

☐ Do we have mutual respect?

☐ Do we communicate well?

☐ Do I feel listened to?

☐ Do I listen?

☐ Do I have confidence in my doctor?

☐ Am I involved with my health?

6

Your Relationship with the Doctor's Staff

*"Patients and their family members have to be nice to
my staff too. My staff are my front line."*

JO ANN C. PULLEN, MD, INTERNAL MEDICINE AND GERIATRICS,
LOS ANGELES, CA

It is important to realize that you don't just have a relationship with your
doctor. Much of your communication is through the office staff. You may
also have quite a bit of interaction with the doctor's nurse, nurse practitioner
or medical assistant, depending on the size or type of practice. Please don't
minimize their importance.

Each doctor's office is different. There may be one assistant who basically
runs the show for the doctor or there may be several doctors who each
have their own medical secretary. Some doctors' offices will have more than
one nurse. Regardless of how your doctor's office is set up, remember one
thing—befriend the doctor's staff. They are the gatekeepers to your doctor.

The Front Office Staff

The front office staff handles your phone calls, takes messages for prescription
refills, arranges your appointments with the doctor and much more. In all
likelihood you will be dealing with the front office staff more often than
your doctor.

You might speak with a receptionist or appointment secretary. Several
doctors said that the gatekeeper of a doctor's office is the receptionist.

Doctors' offices vary, but the person answering the phone, your immediate contact, is the person you must schmooze to get to the next person. Establish a personal relationship with this person. Get her to remember you as a friendly, good patient. This can pay off in how easily you get an appointment or get through to the doctor or the nurse.

Several medical office managers and medical secretaries emphasized the importance of establishing good relationships with the doctor's front office staff and the doctor's nurse because they take information directly to the doctor. They make recommendations to the physician. Each professional said that you will maximize your care if you make the most of these relationships.

Front office staff, such as appointment secretaries and medical secretaries, are generally not registered nurses, nurse practitioners or physician's assistants. Several medical professionals emphasized the importance of not asking for medical advice from them. If you have a medical problem and need advice, ask to speak to the doctor, doctor's nurse, nurse practitioner or physician's assistant.

"Front desk staff in doctors' offices can be very well intended but they are almost never medically trained. Patients should not accept advice from anyone in the front office who isn't a medical professional."

David A. Rapkin, PhD, Clinical and Health Psychologist, Mind-Body Medicine Group, Division of Head and Neck Surgery, UCLA David Geffen School of Medicine, Los Angeles, CA

When you arrive at the doctor's office, be friendly and polite to the front office staff. You want them on your side in case you need them in the future. And you will. When you are in need, you'll be glad that you have been friendly and appreciative of people who helped you. It's about being smart and taking charge of your end of the relationship with these professionals.

You may be wondering why you are being asked to do all this schmoozing when it is you, the patient, who is paying the bill. True enough. However, medical care is not like it used to be. To get what you want out of your medical care, you must present yourself in a way that increases the likelihood of the medical staff going the extra mile for you. You don't have to go overboard. Just think about what I have said regarding doctors and what their jobs are like now. If doctors are very busy, you can bet their staffs are too.

Establish a relationship with at least one person who is part of the office staff and make her your ally. This may be the appointment secretary, medical assistant, doctor's nurse or office manager. This person will recognize your name, your smiling face and the thank-you card you sent her after she squeezed you in for an appointment on a day that was not convenient. Be friendly with her when you are in the doctor's office. Strike up a conversation. Be memorable. Memorize her name, put it in your address book next to the doctor's name and remember her when you send your doctor a Christmas card or holiday gift.

The Doctor's Nurse

Establish a relationship with the doctor's nurse, as she could be the front line for the doctor, depending on how the office is set up. Be friendly and polite to the doctor's nurse. I know several patients who bring gifts to their doctors' nurses to establish a relationship of appreciation and goodwill.

If you are in need, the doctor's nurse will be the one you will talk to if you cannot reach the doctor. This professional can get your prescriptions filled, do in-office tests, do blood work, assist the doctor with exams and more. You also might end up seeing this nurse for an office visit if the doctor isn't available. Treat her as you would the doctor.

Many primary care physicians emphasized the importance of creating a good relationship with the doctor's primary nurse. One family medicine practitioner said that a patient's way in to the doctor is through the doctor's nurse.

The Nurse Practitioner

A nurse practitioner is a registered nurse who has completed advanced nursing education and has extensive clinical training in the diagnosis, management, treatment and prevention of medical conditions. She provides complete physical examinations, diagnoses and is trained to treat medical conditions, order tests and prescribe and manage patient medication. Preventative care and health maintenance are part of her expertise.

"Nurse practitioners spend more time. If there is a serious issue, the patient can ask the nurse practitioner to bring the doctor in to consult."

Shelley Mendelson,
Healthcare Consultant,
West Los Angeles, CA

The Physician's Assistant

A physician's assistant is licensed to practice medicine under the supervision of a licensed physician. The PA has a similar role to a physician and performs physical exams, diagnoses and treats illness and injury, orders and interprets

> "The patient always has the option to see the doctor. There will be less wait time for an appointment with the PA. We spend more time and can be less expensive to hire."
>
> Lauren Fite,
> Physician's Assistant, Los Angeles, CA

tests, encourages preventative health care and in some states can write prescriptions.

The Medical Assistant

A medical assistant performs administrative and clinical tasks to support the work of the doctors and other medical professionals in the office. She helps keep the doctor's office running smoothly. Duties vary by office type, location and size of the practice. She might take your vital signs, administer medications or injections, prepare medical instruments and more.

The Medical Office Manager

This person is responsible for the overall operations of a medical practice. She can plan, coordinate and supervise the delivery of health care. Depending on the size of the medical office, she runs the office, supervises how patients are treated, hires employees, handles the budget and more.

PATIENT CHECKLIST

☐ Do I know who my doctor's gatekeeper is?

☐ Do I know who my doctor's nurse is?

☐ Have I found one person on my doctor's staff who is my ally?

☐ Does my doctor's office have a nurse, nurse practitioner or physician's assistant?

7

Scheduling Tips to Get in to See the Doctor
How to Cut Through the Red Tape

"If you previously called the office and had problems getting an appointment, ask to speak to the practice manager, who may be more sensitive to your needs as a consumer. After all, we doctors work for you. You can take your business elsewhere (and should not be afraid, if severely frustrated, to state this). Patients have gone to other physicians for this and the offending office never knows about it. That won't fix the problem."

DAVID LEE SCHER, MD, FACP, FACC, FHRS, HARRISBURG, PA

Your goal when scheduling an appointment with a doctor is to secure a time that works with your schedule. You'll have more of a chance of reaching that goal if you ingratiate yourself with the appointment scheduler.

The appointment scheduler is dealing with many tasks at once and will appreciate you preparing ahead of time so time is not wasted on the phone. If you aggravate the scheduler, you are less likely to get what you want. Keep in mind that more than likely this person has other calls on hold while she is speaking to you.

Disclose Why You Are You Seeing the Doctor

Know what you need to see the doctor for. Be specific about what you need when speaking with the appointment scheduler. For example: "I need to see the doctor for knee pain from a recent injury. I might need an x-ray." This way, the scheduler can allow enough time for you. If you don't explain all that you are coming in for, she might not allot enough time for what you need. Or the doctor may try to accommodate your needs and be forced to push back other patients, making her late for them.

> "Disclosing everything initially on the phone when you make your appointment improves medical care."
>
> J.C., Patient Advocate, Santa Monica, CA

If this doctor runs a rigid practice and is always on time, you must tell the scheduler exactly what you are coming in for or you may have to come back for another appointment.

What to Do If You Can't Get an Appointment Soon Enough

Even when you are in need and must see a doctor as soon as possible, the unfortunate truth is that some busy doctors may not have time to see you for a month or two. This can be frustrating. There are, however, some strategies to get around this.

Use Your Connections

If you call for an appointment and are told the next appointment is in two months, consider employing a few creative tactics. Use any connection you have to the doctor. If a physician referred you, ask that physician to call the doctor you want to see to get you in sooner. If your own doctor won't do that then tell the medical secretary or receptionist the name of the physician who referred you. If you have an HMO, call your primary care physician first, then the medical group, and then your health insurance plan.

> "When a doctor calls to get an appointment for a patient, mountains move. Doctors have an unspoken rule that they accommodate other doctors, their patients and their families."
>
> Anonymous Doctor's Spouse, Los Angeles, CA

If you have a family member or good friend who is a doctor, use that name or ask that person to put in a call to the doctor you want to see. You can also mention family members or good friends who see this doctor.

Yes, you are being asked to drop names and use them to get in to see the doctor. This is about cultivating familiarity with the person who is scheduling your appointment and using any connections you have. Be sure to thank whoever accommodates your needs and helps you get in to see the doctor sooner.

What to Do If You Don't Have Connections

After sixteen months of chronic pelvic pain, I'd seen eleven doctors. It took a story in a major newspaper to find the doctor who diagnosed and treated me correctly. I had no connection or referrals to get an appointment with her.

I called the front office and was then referred to the doctor's nurse. I was told that the first available appointment was a month from the time I'd called.

I began my campaign. My pleading was sincere because I had been in pain for so long and was desperate. I begged and pleaded not only with the doctor's nurse but with other staff as well. I told each person I spoke to about my chronic pelvic pain, how long it had lasted, how many misdiagnoses I'd had and how many doctors I'd seen.

I asked the nurse and other staff to please put me on a cancellation list. I had every intention of calling back a few days later to check. Later that week, I received a phone call from the surgeon's office, offering me a cancellation the next week. I thanked the person profusely. I wrote down her name.

After seeing Dr. T., my high-resolution dynamic MRI was scheduled for three weeks later. I tried my best to get that MRI moved up but to no avail. Again, I began a campaign. I took cookies to the person who had called me with the cancellation to see Dr. T. I then asked to be put on a cancellation list for the MRI. I got a call a week later that there was an opening the following week. I took flowers to the person who called me.

If you don't have any connections or referrals, here are some tips to help you:

- If you are told you have to wait six weeks to see the doctor, ask to be put on a cancellation list.

- Call back every few days to see if there has been a cancellation. Be polite and friendly. You'll be more memorable if you are. If you can cultivate some familiarity with the scheduler, you'll have a better chance of getting an appointment sooner. Chat with her. Find common ground. Try to establish some sort of personal relationship with her.

- If your medical issue is more urgent and you need to see the doctor much sooner, ask to speak to the doctor's nurse. Explain why you need to see the doctor sooner and ask if you can be accommodated. Be polite and friendly. Demanding to be seen will not help you get what you want.

- If you have seen this doctor before about the same medical issue, you can put in a call to her and ask to see her sooner.

- If you cannot reach a live person to schedule an appointment, leave a message, but keep calling back. Sometimes those messages are not checked for hours.

A Last Resort to Get in to See the Doctor

If you have an urgent need to see your doctor and have tried calling, faxing a note, and leaving messages to talk to her and have not heard back, you can always just show up. It helps to bring someone with you for support if you are going to go this route. It's not a method I recommend but if it's urgent, consider this option.

I flew to Florida to help out my eighty-year-old uncle who had just returned home from a hospital stay and a nursing home stay. He developed MRSA in the nursing home. He had seen his doctor a week earlier and had tests done to see if the MRSA was gone. He was waiting for the test results and the weekend was approaching. He called the doctor's office three times over a period of two days and received no answers and no return call. He had pain in his leg where the MRSA had been and had a few other medical concerns.

I called the doctor's office myself but was unable to get through to a live person. I faxed a note explaining who I was and that my uncle had been trying to get a return call from his doctor about important medical concerns and test results.

The next afternoon, there still was no response to any of our efforts. I told my uncle we were going to drive down to his doctor's office and ask to be seen. We arrived and I spoke to the front office staff. I very politely but firmly explained the situation and said that my uncle had to be seen. Within twenty minutes, my uncle was called into an exam room and was seen by his doctor. I introduced myself to the doctor, asked questions and thanked him for seeing my uncle. My uncle is convinced it was my presence that helped him get in. It may have been, as having a family member with an older patient can definitely help.

Sometimes showing up is the best way if you cannot get any response.

PATIENT CHECKLIST

☐ Did I get an appointment with the doctor soon enough?

☐ Have I explored my options if I need to get in sooner?

☐ Did I ask to be put on a cancellation list?

☐ Did I use my connections?

☐ Did I ask the referring doctor to call the doctor I wish to see?

8

Prepare for Your Doctor Visit

"You'll be less nervous about the doctor visit if you come prepared. Before the visit, think about what you want to get out of the visit. Get the most important complaint out first."

JO ANN C. PULLEN, MD, INTERNAL MEDICINE AND GERIATRICS, LOS ANGELES, CA

No one likes to go to the doctor. It makes us nervous. We may be worried about our health, and the unfamiliar and uncomfortable surroundings don't help. We realize that our medical care is in the hands of someone else and we aren't sure if we trust everyone involved.

Anxiety interferes with our ability to remember things and also with our self-confidence.

Sitting in the exam room, we listen to what is happening outside those four walls and wait. We are anxious over what the doctor might tell us, what tests we might have to undergo, and more. We are dressed in a white cotton gown and can't remember some of our questions for the doctor. We can't seem to summon our self-confidence as a take-charge patient.

> "When you go to see a doctor or are in a medical context, and you are in distress, there is a powerful tendency to be in a dependent state."
>
> David A. Rapkin, PhD,
> Clinical and Health Psychologist,
> Mind-Body Medicine Group,
> Division of Head and Neck
> Surgery, UCLA David Geffen
> School of Medicine,
> Los Angeles, CA

We are asked to leave our identity and control at the door of the exam room. There is a definite power differential between us and the doctor. We are forced to put on a gown, leave our purses and wallets aside, and wait for the physician in a room that certainly was not created with our needs in mind. It's an alien experience sitting in the exam room, and not one that is comfortable for me or any other person I know.

> "Patients often come into doctor's offices and clinics trusting, surrendering of self."
>
> David A. Rapkin, PhD,
> UCLA David Geffen School
> of Medicine, Los Angeles, CA

We are alone with our concerns, and we get the impression that we are alone with our problem—until the doctor walks in. We understand she is pressed for time, so we try to cram everything we want into a very short period of time. We enter into a conversation, are asked questions as we are reporting our symptoms and what is happening with our health, become sidetracked with what the doctor says, and…bingo!… we forget important questions we wanted to ask the doctor.

It's not uncommon to leave a doctor's office and remember an important point of our visit that was not addressed. All because seeing a doctor about medical issues is stressful.

I saw a neurologist for the first time. As we discussed my medical condition and he explained a procedure that could potentially eradicate my pain, I became increasingly hopeful that he would help me. I listened, asked a few questions, and walked out of the office, almost giddy because the treatment he suggested gave me hope.

My mother-in-law asked me the next day exactly what the procedure was and I was unable to answer her question accurately. She asked how long the surgery would be. Whoops. I hadn't asked. She asked if this doctor was going to do an ablation. I told her it was pulsed radio frequency. She asked me, "Does that include burning the nerves?" I didn't know. She also asked about the recuperation.

Some take-charge patient I was.

Before I called the doctor to clarify things, I wrote down my questions, and then wrote down the answers when I spoke to him.

Empowering yourself with the strategies in the next section will help you to take charge of yourself as a patient. Even if you slip up, you can always go back to get your questions answered. The bottom line for you is to feel confident, to understand exactly what is going on with your health and to understand what the doctor proposes to do about it.

In the end, you are the one to evaluate your doctor's suggestions and if they are right for you.

Get Ready for Your Doctor Visit

If you prepare for your doctor's appointment, you will feel more in control, less anxious and more in charge. Bring your health summary.

Prepare Your Health Summary

As a take-charge patient, you'll come prepared to the doctor's appointment as if you were seeing a lawyer or an accountant. You wouldn't meet with your accountant if you didn't have your part of the tax preparation in order. Do the same for your doctor. Approach your appointment as you would a friendly business meeting. Being organized and prepared saves time so you have more of it with your doctor.

Your health summary is your most current health profile. Keep it to about one-half to three-quarters of a page in length. (Also see Chapter 3.)

It includes

- A list of questions

- Your top three medical concerns, in order of importance

- A list of your current of medications, dosages, over-the-counter medications, herbs and supplements. Note any medication changes since the last visit

- A list of your current symptoms

- Your medical journal

- Copies of your test results and reports from other doctors

> "I like it when patients come in with a half- to one-page succinct summary of their medical history, medications, the specific doctors they see and their addresses and phone numbers. This saves me time if I don't have to extract information from a patient. That could take me ten minutes."
>
> Beverly Mikes, MD, FACOG, Obstetrics and Gynecology, Cherry Hill, NJ

Create a List of Questions

As a take-charge patient, you are in collaboration with your doctor and keeping track of your medical concerns and issues supports you as a team player with your doctor.

> "I pay attention to every patient. It is more difficult to get information from patients who ramble. It's easier to focus and concentrate on patients who are direct."
>
> Lawrence S. Miller, MD,
> Clinical Professor,
> UCLA David Geffen School
> of Medicine, Los Angeles, CA

Before you see the doctor, create a list of questions you want to discuss with her. Most doctors emphasized keeping questions specific and focused.

You don't have much time with your doctor, so leave out what your aunt went through and what she told you to do. Write down your questions and the doctor's responses in your medical journal. Or ask your doctor if it is okay with her to record the conversation. Microcassette recorders are inexpensive and most cell phones record. A recording of your conversation with the doctor will be useful for you to review later and to share with loved ones. You must first ask for the doctor's permission to record any conversations.

List Your Top Three Medical Concerns

List your top three medical concerns and prioritize them according to importance and urgency. Many doctors expressed frustration over patients who list ten issues they want to address in one appointment. They explained that some patients do not prioritize their physical concerns and then forget which are the most important until the last few seconds of the office visit. "Doorknob Syndrome" identifies a common problem—patients bringing up very important concerns just as doctors are about to leave the exam room.

Here's why it's so important to list your physical concerns in order of importance. It's very easy to engage in a conversation with a doctor and become sidetracked. You may forget that it was the pain in your stomach that was bothering you the most. It's frustrating to leave the doctor's office only to get into the parking lot and remember a very important medical issue that you forgot to mention. You might have to call the doctor to discuss it and end up playing telephone tag.

If you have more than three medical concerns, be prepared to make another appointment to get them all covered.

Create a List of Your Medications

In your health summary, you should have a list of your medications and their dosages, over-the-counter medications, herbs and supplements. Give a copy to your doctor. It is also important to list hormones, ibuprofen, vitamins, and more. You may think your doctor has an up-to-date list, but in all likelihood, she may not. You must provide this for her.

Has any other doctor you've seen prescribed a medication for you? Write that down. For example: "I saw Dr. Bernstein on November 5, 2011. He prescribed Flexeril 5mg to be taken twice a day."

Describe Your Current Symptoms

Symptoms are not always easy to describe, especially if you haven't thought much about them before your office visit. When my medical condition first started, my doctor asked me where my pain was located. I remember pointing to my lower abdominals and saying, "Here." My doctor asked, "In your bladder? Where?" I didn't know if it was my bladder or someplace else, plus the pain fanned out when it caused muscle spasms.

Below is a diagram of the human body. This might help you to describe the location of symptoms or pain.

Human anatomy

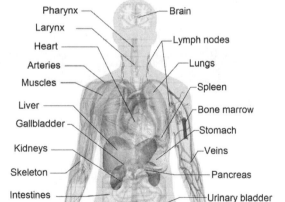

The more detail you can provide to your doctor, the more she can help you. Details become apparent when you observe your symptoms and keep track of them in your medical journal.

Questions to Ask Yourself

- When did I first begin experiencing symptoms?
- Have my symptoms changed over time?
- Does anything make them worse or better?
- How severe are my symptoms?
- Is there pain related to my symptoms?
- Were the symptoms or pain first triggered by a physical event?
- What have I tried to alleviate the symptoms or pain?
- What do I think is causing my symptoms or associated pain?
- If I have pain, how severe is it on a scale of one to ten, one being very mild and ten being very painful?

Describe Your Current Symptoms

If you think about these questions before you see your doctor and jot down some notes in your medical journal, you will be much better prepared to answer your doctor's questions.

If You Have Pain

If you are experiencing pain, it is important to describe the pain in a way that your doctor can understand.

Tips:

- On a scale of one to ten, ten being the worst, how bad is your pain?
- Is the pain the same all the time or does it come and go?
- Is it stabbing pain or a dull ache?
- Is it a knife-like pain or does it radiate? (*Radiate* means it starts at one place and moves, such as moving up your arm or down your leg.)
- Is the pain shooting or throbbing?
- Is the pain debilitating or are you able to carry on?
- What brings on the pain?
- What makes it better?
- When does it tend to come on? Afternoon? Evening? In the middle of the night?

It is very important to describe where the pain is located in your body. Think about this before you see your doctor. Write notes in your medical journal.

Bring Your Medical Journal

If you have not been feeling well, have an ongoing medical condition or a difficult-to-understand set of symptoms, using a notebook to jot down notes on how you are feeling can assist your communication with your physician.

Your medical journal is for keeping track of symptoms, listing questions for your doctor when you think of them, noting research you might have found and more. You can also use it for taking notes on what your doctor tells you during the office visit. Perhaps there is a test your doctor wants you to have by a certain date. Write the information in your medical journal. If your doctor gives you a diagnosis and treatment plan, write them in your medical journal. You will be able to refer to it later.

If you don't feel up to taking notes during your office visit, you can always ask a loved one to do it for you.

Some things to think about:

- How long have I been feeling this way?

- Where is the discomfort or pain located?

- What are the symptoms?

- What have I tried to alleviate the symptoms?

- What makes the symptoms worse or better, such as exercise or eating a meal?

Why Being Prepared for the Doctor Visit Is So Important

If you bring copies of test results ordered by other physicians and a current medication list, your doctor won't have to lasso your information from other sources. If you come

> "The same way we have a dent in our car and we mentally record that when we bring it into the shop to be repaired, make a list of your current symptoms and medical issues that need to be addressed by your physician."
>
> Elizabeth A. Williams, PhD,
> Vanderbilt-Ingram Cancer Center, Nashville, TN

prepared with all the necessary information, you make it easier for your doctor to do her job. She has more time to focus on you. If you come prepared, your doctor will know you are invested in your health just as she is. That in itself contributes to maximizing the medical care you receive.

Not Every Medical Professional in the Office Is a Doctor

Several doctors mentioned that it is important that patients know who they are seeing in the office. They said that sometimes patients will think the physician's assistant or nurse is a doctor. Find out who you are seeing. Not everyone in a doctor's office is a doctor. Ask questions.

PATIENT CHECKLIST

☐ Do I know what I want to get out of the doctor's appointment?

☐ Do I have my list of questions?

☐ Do I have my top three medical concerns?

☐ Do I have my list of medications?

☐ Do I have copies of relevant tests results?

☐ Did I create my health summary?

☐ Do I have a list of current symptoms and do I know how to describe them?

☐ Do I have my medical journal?

☐ Did I ask if I am seeing the doctor or another medical professional in the practice?

9

The Doctor Will See You Now

"Know your primary concern.
If you have chest pain, bring it up first."

JACK C. ROSENFELD, MD, FAMILY MEDICINE, LANSDALE, PA

Here are a few basics about your doctor's appointment that will allow you to maximize the time with her and also keep you on track so you get the most of what your doctor has to offer. You may think you know all of this already but according to doctors and other medical professionals, many patients don't.

Waiting for the doctor is a major complaint from many patients so I'll begin with some information on that.

Wait Time in the Doctor's Office

It's tough to avoid waiting in a doctor's office. Doctors have emergencies that take them away from patients and some of their patients require more time than they were scheduled for. The average time a patient waits for a physician is twenty-two minutes and some waits stretch to an hour or two, according to a 2009 report by Press Ganey Associates, a health care consulting firm.

"Sometimes I plan to be in the office and then I have patients who have emergencies. I can get paged and Mrs. Smith is short of breath. I have to tend to that. Someday you may be Mrs. Smith."

Alan C. Jasper, MD,
Internal Medicine and Pulmonary
Diseases, Los Angeles, CA

Tips to Cut Wait Time in the Doctor's Office

- Schedule the doctor's first appointment in the morning or the first after lunch.

- Complete paperwork in advance.

- Make sure all of your test results are in the doctor's office in advance of your appointment.

- Call forty-five minutes before your appointment and ask if the doctor is running on time.

- Before you go to your appointment, make sure your insurance covers it. Call your insurance company and ask questions.

- Ask the front desk person when you make your appointment if the doctor double books patients. Ask this person how long you may have to wait if she double books.

Don't Complain If Your Doctor Has Squeezed You In

If you have requested a same-day appointment with your doctor, and she has squeezed you in, don't complain if you have to wait. She has done you a favor by fitting you in on a day she was not expecting you. Be grateful and patient.

Too many doctors told me about patients who are sick and are squeezed in on the same day and complain to the office staff about the amount of time they had to wait.

Now, it's legitimate to be upset if you have a previously scheduled appointment and you are forced to wait two hours to see the doctor. But if the doctor's staff has done you a favor because you are very sick or have an urgent problem, you aren't going to get what you want if you complain. One doctor reported finding it difficult to respond in the way he would like to patients in this situation. It creates tension and resentment if you complain after the doctor has done you a favor. Be smart about this. You want the best medical care.

How to Maximize Your Time with Your Doctor

As a patient, you must realize that you will have to answer questions about your health when you see your doctor. To get the most out of the visit, write down the answers to the following questions before you meet with your doctor:

- Has something changed since my last visit?
- When did it change?
- How long has it been this way?
- When do I most notice the symptoms?
- Does anything make the symptoms worse or better?
- Has my medication changed since my last visit?
- Did I have a test or procedure? If so, did I bring a copy of the results?

Know Why You Are Seeing the Doctor

Believe it or not, several doctors told me stories about patients who arrived in their offices and had no idea why they were there. More than likely, these patients did not ask their primary care physicians why they were being referred to specialists.

This may seem like it goes without saying, but know why you are seeing a doctor and ask why a doctor has referred you to another doctor.

Be on Time for Your Doctor's Appointment

If you are late to a doctor's appointment, not only will you risk not having enough time for your visit, but this will also push back other patients and force the office staff to reorganize the doctor's time. This is not a good way to ingratiate yourself to anyone in the doctor's office. You may need them in the future.

This is about being a smart patient so you get the best medical care. Be on time, polite and friendly. You want the doctor's staff on your side.

Get Blood Work Done ahead of Time

Get blood work done ahead of time whenever possible so the doctor can look at the results and discuss them with you in person. This prevents the need for a phone call a week later. This way, everything is current when you see the doctor.

Bring Copies of Tests Ordered by Other Doctors

If you have seen other doctors who ordered tests, bring copies of the results with you. Bring copies of MRIs, CT scans, reports from procedures, etc., to this doctor. You want to make the most of your doctor's time. You don't want her using it to gather your medical information from elsewhere.

Orient Your Physician

Remind the doctor in the current appointment where you left off in the previous appointment. She has seen many other patients since the last time she saw you, and it's unlikely that she'll remember every detail of your last appointment. For example you can say, "The last time I saw you, we discussed x." Or, "I talked to you on the phone about x, y, and z."

Present Your Health Summary to Your Doctor

Chapter 3 explains all you need to know about creating your health summary. Here are a few of the main points.

Your health summary includes

- your contact information;
- names of doctors you were referred to and reports from those doctors;
- insurance company;
- your top three medical concerns;
- your symptoms and changes in your health;
- diagnoses you have received;
- copies of any test results since you last saw this doctor;
- your list of medications and dosages;
- any changes in medications or new medications;
- your list of questions for the doctor.

Disclose Your Health History

Most doctors emphasized the importance of disclosing your health history. This includes sexual history, habits, drug history, past medical conditions, current medical conditions and anything else that could affect your health.

Be Honest with Your Doctor

Most doctors said that it is extremely important for patients to be honest with them. They are not in the judgment business. Your doctor needs to know the truth about you, your health and your lifestyle so she can help you. If you lie or hide something from your doctor, you are only hurting yourself. You might be doing something or taking something that could interfere with a medical treatment your doctor has given you. Keep her informed.

If you use drugs or have in the past, tell your doctor. If you smoke, tell your doctor. Sometimes people don't realize that these behaviors can affect what a doctor prescribes for you now.

Tell her what she needs to know so she can do her job.

"I had a patient come in with vague complaints-joint pain, weakness, fatigue. He left out the germane history, that he had served in Vietnam and when he and his friends were bored they would inject heroin. He had contracted hepatitis C through this practice. It took quite some time to order tests, to diagnose hepatitis C, as the history was somewhat incomplete. It then took even longer for him to tell me when he may have been inoculated with the hepatitis C virus, and to develop a treatment plan. He was also somewhat lackadaisical with his appointments, as well as avoiding liver toxins. 'You have to educate yourself, and assume some responsibility for your own care' I told him. 'You can't just wait for a liver transplant.' He soon started to keep appointments with the hepatologists. He often read about the disease and started to intervene and take care of himself."

Alan Bailer, DO, Internal Medicine, Cheltenham, PA

Know What Your Health Insurance Plan Covers

Whether you are going to your doctor for a sick visit or well visit (preventative care visit), ask your insurance company ahead of time if it will be covering the cost, how much of the cost it will cover and what your co-pay is.

Understand Your Diagnosis

It is imperative that you understand your diagnosis. When you meet with your doctor, bring your medical journal and write everything down.

Questions to Ask Your Doctor about Your Diagnosis:

- What is my diagnosis?
- Where can I find information about my diagnosis? Do you have information you can give me?
- Are there any other possible diagnoses for my condition?
- What do I need to do to recover?
- How long do you think it will take for me to recover?
- What tests and procedures do I need to have done?
- Are there alternatives to these tests and procedures?
- What changes do I need to make to support my recovery?
- Do I need another appointment with you?

Before your appointment, write all these questions down in your medical journal. Be sure to write down the answers during or after your appointment. We all have trouble remembering what doctors tell us. You will be able to refer to your notes later.

Resist Diagnosing Yourself

Don't come in with your own diagnosis after researching your symptoms on the internet. You can bring in some research from credible websites and ask questions, but allow your doctor to make her own diagnosis.

Try not to interpret your symptoms—simply describe them. If you begin the conversation with, "I think I have bronchitis," you're not allowing the doctor to diagnose you. You can phrase it like this instead, "I have been coughing for over a week and still have a fever."

Understand Your Treatment Plan

Sometimes we can walk away from a doctor's office and realize we are not clear about what the doctor wants us to do. This is understandable, because as we converse with the doctor, we can get sidetracked and forget important details. It's important to prepare ahead of time so this won't happen to you.

Sample questions about treatment plans:

- What is my treatment plan?
- What will I have to do?
- I'm writing all of this down, but do you have a sheet with instructions?
- How long will it take for me to feel better?
- How long will I have to follow this treatment plan?

When presented with a treatment plan, you must decide whether you can follow what the doctor is suggesting. If you can't follow her recommendations, you must tell her why. Whether it is because you cannot afford the medications, procedures, physical therapy or whatever it is or your lifestyle cannot accommodate what she suggests, you must tell her. This way, she knows how to work with you and can offer alternatives. It's not "her way or the highway" every single time. As a take-charge patient, you work in collaboration with your doctor.

Doctors want to know if you understand what they are suggesting to you and they want to know if you will comply with the treatment plan they recommend. They want to hear from you if a medication isn't working or if you didn't see the specialist they recommended and why.

Doctors are your partners in your medical care. They are not dictators, gods or parents. You must do your part and be proactive in your care.

Follow Your Prescribed Treatment Plan

A take-charge patient follows her doctor's instructions and if she cannot, she takes the initiative to explain what prevents her from doing so.

Perhaps you feel the treatment plan isn't working, or there are unpleasant side effects or you cannot follow through for some other reason. Tell the doctor! She can come up with alternatives that might better suit you or she may simply reassure you that you need to give the treatment a few more days to work. Either response is very important.

A passive patient is one who does not follow doctors' instructions and drops the ball. This compromises her health and medical care.

Understand Your Medications

If your doctor prescribes a medication for you, don't pocket the prescription without asking questions. Studies confirm that if patients know more about medications they are prescribed, they are more apt to take them.

Not that I haven't done this myself, but later I had to call my pharmacist and research the medication to find out what I needed to know.

Sample Questions about Medications:

- What is the name of the medication? Would you please give me the brand and generic names of the medication you are prescribing?

    This keeps you informed if you receive the medication at the pharmacy and it has a different name.

- How many times a day do I take it?

- Do I need to take it with food?

- Is this medication to treat the diagnosis you gave me?

- How long will I be on the medication?

"Patients must level with their doctor if they are unable to follow his/her orders and they should explain why. For example, if the doctor gives the patient an exercise prescription and instructs him to walk five days a week and if the patient is unable to comply, he must be honest with the doctor about why he can't comply. He may complain of fatigue with exercise in which case the doctor will investigate the cause of his fatigue. Another example is if the doctor puts a patient on a low sodium diet and the patient doesn't follow the instruction, he should level with the physician about why he could not comply. He may have craved high sodium foods or may eat out frequently. The doctor can then review the diet with the patient and change it to suit the patient's lifestyle or review the sodium content of foods the patient likes and tell the patient which foods are better."

Alan E. Karz, MD,
Cardiology, Valencia, CA

Remember, do not stop a medication without informing your doctor. If you leave a message and do not get a return phone call within two days, call back and ask that the doctor call you as soon as possible.

Understand Your Tests and Procedures

Undergoing tests and procedures can be frightening. To gain confidence and feel less frightened, ask as many questions as you can about the test or procedure so you are more knowledgeable about it. Ask your doctor for written information about the test or procedure.

Sample Questions:

- What is the procedure/test?
- What are you looking for?
- How long will it take?
- Will I be able to drive afterward?
- Do I have to prepare for this procedure/test?
- Will I be able to go back to work right afterward?

If you see your doctor with symptoms and she doesn't find a reason for your symptoms, you can ask if you should have a test. Yes, you can ask if you need a test. Be assertive.

"A female patient came in complaining of abdominal pain. She also suffered from an anxiety disorder so the doctor became desensitized to her consistent complaints of pain and wrote them off to her anxiety disorder. The patient persisted and asked the doctor to keep searching for the cause of her abdominal pain. Reluctantly, her gastroenterologist agreed to do a colonoscopy which revealed large pre-cancerous colon nodules which had to be surgically removed. Had the patient not persisted, the nodules would have become cancerous and could have spread throughout her colon."

Anonymous Medical Secretary, Miami, FL

Follow Through with Tests and Procedures

If your doctor recommends that you have a test such as a colonoscopy, be sure that you do it. No one likes to have them, but as a responsible patient, you must. Just make the appointment and get it over with. Ask for the report to be sent to your doctor's office and get a copy for yourself. Bring it to your next appointment with your PCP just in case she has not received it.

Ask for Your Test Results

If your doctor does any kind of test and you haven't received the results within a week or two, call and ask for them. Research shows that no news isn't necessarily good news. You must call your doctor's office and ask for the results and discuss them with your doctor. Request that a copy of the results be mailed, emailed or faxed to you. Place it in your health file.

A study published in the *Annals of Internal Medicine* examined the medical records of more than 2,500 patients and found that doctors didn't always know about test results that red-flagged a serious problem. If your doctor has done blood work, an MRI, CT scan or any other kind of test, call her office and ask for the results. It could be that the doctor missed it. Get your results!

Your Annual Checkup

Your annual checkup is extremely important. Several doctors emphasized the importance of a yearly physical. Whether you see a primary care physician or a specialist who doubles as a PCP, your doctor needs a yearly baseline for you and your health. Some doctors said that it is not fair to the doctor to simply see her when you are sick because she will have nothing to compare your current condition to.

"Don't wait for a routine office visit to address your ongoing problems."

Beverly Mikes, MD, FACOG,
Obstetrics and Gynecology,
Mt. Laurel, NJ

Make a list of questions for your doctor before your annual physical. Ask yourself what you want out of the visit. For example, "I want to know if I am healthy" or "I'm reaching a milestone age and I want to know which tests I need to have."

Several doctors admitted to finding it objectionable if a patient calls for advice and she has not been seen for two years. If you need advice on a medical condition and your doctor has not recently seen you, make an appointment. Doctors don't get paid for phone calls, nor do they get paid for emails. Many doctors will not refill a prescription if you have not seen them for six months.

The Importance of Following Up with the Doctor

You may not realize just how important it is to follow up with your doctor. You are in a partnership with your doctor about your health and you must do your part. You might not want to go back, especially if you feel better, but if the doctor has asked you to schedule a follow-up visit with her, show up! This is your responsibility. If you want the best care, you have to follow through.

> *"I had a female patient in her early fifties who had a growth on her face. I wanted to biopsy it. I squeezed the patient in the very next day for a biopsy and the patient didn't show up. Despite my calling her and expressing concern that the growth was abnormal and a possible skin cancer, the patient didn't come in. She waited one and a half years to come back. The growth proved to be skin cancer on her nose. She now needed reconstruction."*
>
> Molly Griffin, MD, Dermatology, Los Angeles, CA

Speak Up and Ask Questions!

Many patients are afraid to ask questions of their doctors. It's okay to feel this way but you must understand what your doctor is telling you about your medical condition, disease or treatment plan. If you don't, you may not comply with her treatment plan and you will not get better.

If you do not understand the medical jargon your doctor is using, ask her to explain. I have done this several times with different doctors. I simply say, "I don't understand what that term means. Can you please explain?" And every time each doctor has explained.

Years ago, I did feel a little sheepish about asking questions but I don't anymore. I got used to it. It's like exercising a muscle. Use it and it gets stronger.

If you don't think you can digest everything the doctor will tell you, bring a loved one with you to take notes. You can discuss the information with this person after the appointment to clarify details.

After Your Visit with Your Doctor

Here are some things to think about after you have seen your doctor.

- Did I feel comfortable with my doctor?

- Did I get all my questions answered?

- Do I feel comfortable with the diagnosis she gave me? Do I agree with the doctor's diagnosis and treatment plan?

- Do I understand what the doctor told me?

- Do I understand what the doctor wants me to do?

- If I received a prescription for a medication, do I know what the name of the medication is, what it is for and when I am supposed to take it?

- If I am to have a procedure, do I know the name of the procedure, what it is, what it is for, what I need to do to prepare for it, and what I need to do following it?

- Do I feel comfortable following the doctor's recommendations?

- Do I need a second opinion?

PATIENT CHECKLIST

- ☐ Do I know why I am seeing the doctor?

- ☐ Did we discuss any tests she requested?

- ☐ Did we discuss information from other doctors I've seen?

- ☐ Do I understand my diagnosis and treatment plan?

- ☐ Do I understand any new medications the doctor prescribed?

- ☐ Can I follow the prescribed treatment plan?

10

Specialists

"If a particular concern is noted, your primary care physician should refer you to a specialist; you or your caregiver can also make a specialist appointment directly. If the concern is the result of a test, make sure that test (not just the report) is transmitted to the specialist or brought with you at the visit. Failure to do so may result in a wasted trip. If the referral is by another physician, make sure the reason for the referral is clear to you. This will help start a better discussion with the specialist at the beginning of the visit."

DAVID LEE SCHER, MD, FACP, FACC, FHRS,
HARRISBURG, PA

What Is a Specialist?

A specialist is a medical doctor who has advanced training and experience in identifying and treating diseases and conditions of particular parts of the body. For example, a cardiologist treats conditions related to the heart.

Specialists tend to focus on their specialty and not on the whole picture. For example, if you have lung problems, the pulmonologist may focus only on your lungs and not on related parts of your body.

How to Find Specialists

If you need to see a specialist and you have not already been referred to one by your primary care physician, ask another doctor whom you trust.

> "You don't want to see a specialist I don't know. We all see each other at the hospital, at meetings, social events, the doctors' parking lot. We all communicate formally and informally."
>
> Jo Ann C. Pullen, MD,
> Internal Medicine and
> Geriatrics, Los Angeles, CA

As said before, good doctors generally refer to other good doctors.

Some say that doctors refer to their buddies, and that is true in some cases, but you have to start somewhere. Plus, doctors choose other doctors for you to see whom they trust. Most choose doctors who will communicate with them about patients.

Most doctors agreed that they prefer patients to see doctors they work with because they have experience with these doctors, communicate with them more often and have established relationships with them. They know their track records from other patients they've sent to them.

On the other hand, medical office managers and nurses did mention that some doctors refer patients to their friends regardless of how much they know about what kind of care the specialists provide. Just something to keep in mind as you do your research on doctors you may want to see.

Tips to Find a Specialist:

- Start with one doctor you think is very good. Ask her for a referral to a specialist.

- Ask your primary care physician for a referral to a specialist.

- Talk to your family and friends and find out if they have seen specialists they respect and like.

- Call an emergency room registered nurse and ask if she knows a good specialist for what you need. These nurses see doctors in action and they know who responds to pages and who visits patients in the hospital.

- If you have a chronic medical condition or serious illness, start by asking your primary care physician or other physician you trust for a specialist who is affiliated with a highly respected medical school and specializes in your medical condition, injury or disease.

- Research each doctor. For more information on how to do research, see Chapter 13.

Find Specialists Affiliated with Your Hospital

Many of the doctors I interviewed recommended that you see doctors who are affiliated with the hospital of your choice. Imagine if you have a gall bladder issue and you see a gastroenterologist who is not affiliated with the hospital you prefer. If you have a serious gastrointestinal issue that requires hospitalization, then you will not be seen by your doctor.

What to Do If You See a Specialist Your PCP Does Not Know

The time to seek out a specialist who may not be part of your PCP's network is when you need a doctor who is very experienced in your medical condition, when you have conflicting diagnoses, or when you have a serious medical condition and your research leads you to a specialist at a major medical institution.

If you have a problem that has either been misdiagnosed or is a serious or complicated medical issue, or if you have no diagnosis at all, most doctors and other medical professionals agree—go to a doctor affiliated with a major medical institution and who specializes in your medical condition.

One drawback to seeing a specialist who is not connected to your PCP is that your doctor has no connection or experience with this specialist. You are basically starting from scratch.

If You See a Big Name Specialist

It's easy to put full faith in a doctor you've heard or read a lot about. Just because this doctor is well known in the community or around the globe, you can't forget all the strategies in this book. When we meet with someone who is respected not only by peers but by others as well, we can easily allow ourselves to become disempowered. Although this doctor may be revered, she is not superhuman. She is a working professional just like the others. Come prepared to the office visit, engage in the conversation and ask questions. Several doctors said to make sure you get second and even third opinions even if you have already seen a highly respected specialist.

Your Relationship with the Specialist

If you have found the best doctor for your particular condition, you might have to accept character you have carefully screened out with your choice of PCP or internist.

I'll give you an example. I saw a specialist for my ongoing chronic medical condition. I believe he is a very good doctor. However, he did not return my phone calls—his nurse always did. He was not the type of doctor who worked in partnership with me as a take-charge patient. He was cordial, very intelligent and educated. But I never got the impression that he was eager to discuss my condition in collaboration with me as his patient. He explained things well but very briefly. His demeanor didn't welcome my participation or questions about my care.

> "Sometimes you make the trade-off between a good technician and someone who is more caring and aware of the importance of dealing with pain—because sometimes what is most important is to have a good plumber."
>
> Cheri Adrian, PhD, Clinical Psychologist, Los Angeles, CA

It was the nurse who called me back with test results, answers to my questions or prescriptions to treat my condition. Sometimes there was miscommunication because she was the go-between. More than once, I had to ask her to ask the correct question of the doctor. This doctor was simply too busy and saw too many patients in a day.

If You Can't Get an Appointment with a Specialist

If you are having trouble getting an appointment soon enough with a specialist you haven't seen before, call your referring doctor. Ask if she can help you by calling the doctor herself. If that is not possible, use your connections. Do you know any physicians who are friends with this doctor? Do you know any patients who see this doctor? Mention their names. You want to create a sense of familiarity with the doctor's front desk person by dropping names and using connections.

When you are in need, you don't want to wait a month or two to see a doctor if you can help it.

Ask to be put on a cancellation list. Provide all of your contact information so if an appointment opens up, the scheduler will be able to reach you immediately. She is not going to hold onto that appointment for long if she can't reach you. Other patients want that appointment too. Call back every few days and speak to the same person. Ask if there have been any cancellations. Charm the scheduler. Be friendly and polite. This will help her to remember you.

I did not have any connections to Dr. T., the surgeon who cured me of sixteen months of chronic pelvic pain. No doctor referred me to her and I knew no one who had ever seen her before. I was told when I called that I would have to wait a month to see her. I asked to be put on a cancellation list. I told the scheduler my sad story (all true) and shared how desperate I was to get in to see Dr. T. A few days later, I was called with a cancellation.

The Value of Getting a Second Opinion

Several doctors emphasized the importance of getting second and even third opinions even if you have seen a specialist who has recommended a certain medical treatment. No matter how much you've heard about how great a specialist is, still get a second opinion.

As a take-charge patient you must trust your gut instincts. You know that a recommended test, treatment or surgery might be the perfect recommendation but you also know that you must research each doctor and each suggested treatment for what ails you. This might include a second opinion, especially if what the doctor recommends doesn't feel right, doesn't make sense or if your research leads you to another option.

As one physician said in regard to specialists, "Remember, when you are a hammer, everything looks like a nail."

"Carol is a seventy-six-year old patient living in Los Angeles. She was in excellent health and walked one to two miles a day. One day she experienced sudden and severe low back pain and went to see her primary care physician. He examined her and said he thought the back pain would go away on its own and suggested she come back to see him if it didn't in a week or two.

Carol used a heating pad to lessen the pain. Per her doctor's instructions, she limited her activity, avoiding stretching and heavy lifting. The pain persisted and one week later she paid another visit to her doctor. He ordered x-rays of her lower back.

The radiologist saw a lump on her x-rays. Carol's primary care doctor called her and explained that a lump was visible on the films. At that moment, Carol was shocked, unable to think straight, and simply forgot to ask all the necessary questions. Her primary care doctor suggested she repeat the x-rays in three months.

Carol was frightened. She said, "I didn't feel comfortable with waiting three months for a follow-up." The next morning, she called her primary care doctor and asked to be referred to a specialist to discuss the lump and her options.

Carol was then referred to a pulmonary specialist. She had her x-rays and radiologist's written reports with her. The pulmonologist examined her, and looked at her records and told her she was in good health. He agreed with her primary care physician that she should simply follow up in three months with repeat x-rays. Carol told him she wasn't comfortable with taking a "wait and see" approach for three months. She asked if he could biopsy the lump. The pulmonologist told her that she could not have a biopsy because the lump in her rib area was inaccessible.

Carol returned home upset and anxious. She couldn't sleep. She was not an assertive person with medical professionals, but decided to call the pulmonologist the next morning. She politely told him that she wanted take the necessary steps to find out what the lump was. She was referred to a thoracic surgeon at a major teaching hospital.

Carol had immediate rapport with the thoracic surgeon. After looking at her x-rays, he told her she had a tumor in her lung. This was the first she had heard of that. The surgeon told her that even though the tumor may be benign, it didn't belong there and recommended that she have it removed. Carol had the surgery within ten days of the office visit with the thoracic surgeon and the entire tumor was removed. The pathology report showed the tumor was malignant, but luckily it had not spread. Her prognosis was excellent.

As of today, Carol has been cancer free for five years."

Sister of the Patient, Los Angeles, CA

Second Opinions Online

Several world-renowned hospitals currently offer online second opinions to patients. Two of them are Cleveland Clinic and Partners Online Specialty Consultations, which is affiliated with Massachusetts General Hospital.

Online consultations are sometimes the only option you have. Some doctors frown on them because the doctor is limited: she cannot examine you, is not in the room to evaluate you, and cannot fully assess you as a patient. However, if you don't have access to doctors at a major, world-class teaching hospital, this could be a very viable option.

Tips on Using Online Second Opinions:

- Insurance may not pay for online consultations. Call your health insurance company and ask questions. If this type of consultation is not covered, ask for the cost ahead of time.

- At the time of this printing, these are the costs:

  ○ Cleveland Clinic charges $565 for an online second opinion. If a pathologist is necessary, there is an additional cost of $185.

  ○ Partners Online Specialty Consultations charges $495 for an online second opinion. If a radiologist is necessary they charge an additional $200 and if a pathologist is necessary, an additional $250.

- Prepare your questions ahead of time. Enlist a family member or good friend who can help you create concise and very specific questions you need answered.

- Ahead of time, supply the doctor with copies of your records, reports from your doctors, test results and copies of MRIs, CT scans, x-rays, etc.

- Take notes during the consultation.

- Refer to your written questions.

- If you would like a loved one to be present during the consultation to act as a second set of eyes and ears, ask for permission from the doctor ahead of time.

Your Appointment with the Specialist

"I had a patient who came to me for a second opinion. This patient belonged to Kaiser. He came to see me and was accompanied by his wife and son. He did not bring any medical records and had minimal information and recollection about his previous medical history. This patient was demanding. What he wanted from me was unfair and unrealistic. I can't help much when I have no medical records from a patient, don't know which tests were done, and know little about the patient's medications and history."

Daniel Wohlgelernter, MD, Cardiology, Santa Monica, CA

Before you go to an office visit with a doctor for a second opinion, please be sure you do the following:

- Collect copies of your most recent tests, scans and reports on your current medical condition.

- Research your current medical condition and take notes in your medical journal.

- Create a list of questions for the doctor.

Ask the specialist to send a report to your primary care physician. Also get a copy of the report for yourself.

If the second opinion contradicts the first, you might consider going for a third opinion from another doctor.

If You See a Managed Care Specialist

If you are referred to a doctor by a Health Maintenance Organization (HMO) and not by your primary physician, it is especially important that you come to the office prepared, as you may have no connection to this doctor other than your HMO.

Your HMO can decide where you go to get, for example, an angiogram. You must get two copies of the angiogram report so that you can present one to your primary care physician and place one in your health file.

*"If you have an HMO or managed care and are restricted to
seeing in-network doctors, spend the money to find a competent
expert in your disease or condition and get a second opinion
outside of your insurance company. Have this expert give you
his/her diagnosis and a list of necessary tests. This expert can
send your HMO/managed care doctor a consultation with his/
her diagnosis and recommended tests. The patient can have
their HMO/managed care doctor order the tests in network to
minimize cost to the patient."*

Lawrence S. Miller, MD, Clinical Professor,
UCLA David Geffen School of Medicine,
Los Angeles, CA

When a physician recommends surgery, tests, or a certain treatment
plan, try to remember not to rush your decision to go ahead unless it is
medically necessary. Trust your instincts. If you aren't sure about what the
doctor is recommending, get a second opinion.

Sometimes patients will rush into treatment because they are afraid,
want to move quickly or because they are in pain and want it to end. Take
the time to find a qualified doctor and get a second opinion.

Tips to Prevent Fragmented Care

If you are seeing multiple doctors or are going to multiple medical
institutions, there is likely to be a breakdown in communication. By doing
what is suggested below you can help prevent it.

You can help the specialists see you as a whole person by presenting a
complete picture of your medical situation. Orient them every time you meet
with them. Let them know what other physicians are doing with your care.

Bring Copies of Your Records to Each Doctor

Bring copies of pertinent records from your PCP and other specialists you've
seen. Include a very brief description of what occurred in each previous
visit, the date you saw each doctor, and results of tests, scans, and reports
about your current medical condition.

Bring a List of Your Medications

> "If you go to several doctors, bring your list of medications, dosages, and which doctors prescribed them."
>
> Joseph J. Morgan, MD, President,
> Pharmaceutical Industry Consultants,
> Yardley, PA

Bring a list of your current medications, dosages, allergies to medications, over-the-counter medications, herbs and supplements.

Several doctors suggested bringing the bottles of medicine with you for them to take a look at.

Prepare a List of Questions Ahead of Time

In your medical journal, create a list of questions for each doctor ahead of time. Write down the answers. You might be able to record the conversation with the doctor, but you must first ask permission. Any kind of record will help you keep information straight.

Take Notes on Each Visit with Your Doctor

Take notes on conversations with your doctors. This is to help you remember what each doctor said. You can refer to your notes later and go over them with a trusted loved one or another doctor. This will help you remember what medical condition you have, what new tests your doctor wants you to have, what new specialists your doctor wants you to see and what new medications were prescribed.

Obtain Copies of Your Medical Records at Each Medical Encounter

Ask for copies of your records at each doctor visit. You don't need your entire chart. If you end up getting more than you need, simply sift through the documents and keep what you think is relevant to your current medical issue.

Facilitate Communication between Your Doctors

If you request your doctors to talk to one another, be sure that each one has the other's contact information. You might have to provide written permission for each doctor to speak to the other about you.

If you learn that your doctors haven't talked, you can follow up by emailing or faxing each doctor. You can write, "Thank you for seeing me on (date). I enjoyed meeting you. Just a friendly reminder to please contact

Dr. X about my (name of medical condition)." Include Dr. X's contact information so all she has to do is look at your fax and call the other doctor.

> "Patients have this idea that doctors all talk to one another all the time. It just doesn't happen."
>
> Anonymous MD, Cardiology,
> Los Angeles, CA

You are making this easy for your doctor because you want the task completed in a timely manner. This is for your benefit.

What to Do If Your Doctor Drops the Ball

If the communication between your doctors still has not occurred, call the office of the physician who hasn't initiated the necessary communication. Speak to her nurse or office manager and explain the situation. Let her know that you made the request and provide the other doctor's contact information. Ask for her help. You can also say, "I don't want to be a pest, but Dr. X is awaiting her call." If this nurse actually gets the job done and your doctor completes the communication, consider mailing a simple thank you note to reinforce your appreciation. This will help identify you as a nice patient should you ever need her help again.

You are trying to make this as easy as possible for all the doctors involved so you get more out of your medical care.

It can be frustrating when your doctors do not communicate with one another when they said they would. You can spend time and energy on getting angry with them or you can channel that energy toward facilitating progress. Consider saving complaints for things that are really important such as patient neglect, medical errors or egregious errors that could cause you harm.

If you can do one extra thing to support the doctor so that she performs the task, then do it. This is your medical care we are talking about. Do what you have to do to get the job done.

Remember the goal: to get the best medical care possible for you.

How to Sift Through Multiple Medical Opinions

When there are several different opinions from doctors, it's easy to get confused, frustrated or overwhelmed. The opinions may all come from qualified doctors and you may not know what to do or which recommendation to go with. If you have seen two specialists who disagree, do not hesitate to get a third opinion. This third opinion might help you with your decision or confirm one of the other two. If the third opinion does not confirm one of the first two, talk to your primary care physician. Show her your records from these specialists and ask for her opinion.

Here are some suggestions to help you sift through multiple medical opinions:

- Talk with your primary care physician. Make sure you give her all of the other doctors' reports either by email, fax or mail and check to make sure she has received all that she needs. Once she has received the necessary information, call her office and set a time for a phone or office consult. Ask her opinion about which avenue she feels is best for you.

- Do your own research on the opinions from each doctor. Which one makes sense to you?

- Talk to one of the specialists you trust and show her all of the information you have gathered from the other doctors and your own research. Ask her opinion.

- Seek out a specialist from a highly respected medical institution who specializes in the problem you have. If you cannot travel to her location, ask if you can have a consult by phone, Skype™, or some other form of video communication. Before the consultation, provide this doctor with your pertinent medical records. Call three days before your consultation to make sure she has received them.

- Talk to loved ones about what each doctor has said. Show them the reports and try to digest the information with their input.

- Use your instincts. What is logical? What makes sense? Which doctor do you have the most confidence in? Write it down if that helps you.

- If you are connected to medically savvy friends on Facebook, Twitter or other forms of social media, ask them questions.

- Find a medical society or health/medical organization that focuses on your medical condition and search its website for information. See if it has support groups for people with your condition. Support groups are beneficial because you can share information and check out the doctors' opinions you've received with other patients in that group.

And on the other hand…

"To decide which option is best, don't keep getting more opinions. It's too confusing. The patient has to judge the doctors. Evaluate which doctor's answers make the most sense. Ask yourself, which doctor's reasons are the most compelling? When your first and second opinion doctors don't agree, the third doctor may be the tie breaker."

Daniel Wohlgelernter, MD, Cardiology, Santa Monica, CA

Medical Information Overload

You might suffer medical information overload if you have been seeing doctors, researching your medical condition and talking to others about it. It happened to me several times during my chronic medical condition, which lasted sixteen months. There were times when I had simply taken in too much information and I could no longer think straight about any of it.

If this happens, simply take a break and get your mind off all of the information. Do something fun. Sleep. Once you feel refreshed, do some more detective work.

Rural Communities

If you live in a rural community, you may have trouble gaining access to good specialists. Physicians tend to gravitate toward metropolitan areas where the highly respected medical institutions are located.

"My biggest obstacle is that my patients don't have accessibility to specialists. In Southern Maryland there is a physician shortage. Some of my patients have to travel 40 minutes to see a doctor in Washington D.C. or to a doctor in Baltimore, MD. This is difficult for patients with chronic illnesses who have to travel multiple times to specialists who are that far away."

Karlene Ross, MD, Family Medicine, Waldorf, MD

If You Can Travel to a Bigger City

- Ask your primary care physician for her suggestions on how to get to a specialist who can help you with your condition. Ask her if she knows anyone in a larger metropolitan area. If so, she might be able to help you get in to see this professional.

- If your PCP does not know of a specialist to help you, you must do your research on your own. Start by asking friends, family members and colleagues if they know of a specialist who might help you. You can ask, "Do you know of anyone with my medical condition? Who did they see? Was their treatment successful?"

- You can also ask physicians you know for referrals to a top specialist.

- Another option is to find people in online forums and groups with your medical condition and ask which doctors they see and have been successfully treated by.

- You can also go to websites maintained by major medical schools and search for your illness, disease or injury. You will find a list of doctors who specialize in treating what you have.

   Research each doctor and find one or two who have performed the most treatments on the most patients with your medical condition. You might also consider doctors who are on the cutting edge of research.

Once you have names of several specialists, do the following:

- Look up the specialists of your choice on the American Medical Association website and search for board certification in their specialties.

- Call the doctors' offices and gather information. Ask for the doctor's nurse. Explain that you will be traveling from another city to see this doctor. Ask if a copy of the doctor's CV, publications and links to her research could be sent to you.

- Ask questions such as, "I live in (city and state). My doctor here is not able to help with my medical condition. She has given me (diagnosis) or "She has been unable to make a firm diagnosis. My symptoms are.… Is Dr. X the specialist I should see?"

Then call or make an appointment with your PCP and go over the information you have uncovered. Ask for her opinion on which doctor to see.

If You Are Unable to Travel

- Follow all the tips above but request a consultation by phone, Skype™ or some other form of video communication.

- Send copies of your pertinent medical records to this doctor before your appointment.

- Call three days before your appointment and make sure your records have been received. There is nothing worse than planning for an appointment and realizing too late that the doctor never received your records. There is nothing that doctor can do for you unless she has your information and medical history.

  ○ Prepare questions you want to ask ahead of time.

  ○ Take notes during the conversation.

PATIENT CHECKLIST

☐ Have I found referrals for specialists through trusted doctors, loved ones, online forums or groups, medical institution websites or registered nurses at the ER of my local hospital?

☐ Is the specialist affiliated with the hospital of my choice?

☐ Do I need a second opinion?

☐ Have I prepared for my appointment with the specialist? (Do I have copies of pertinent medical records, my health summary, a list of medications and allergies to medications, etc.?)

☐ Have I created a list of questions?

☐ Is my medical journal up to date?

11

How to Prevent Medication Errors and Manage Your Medications

"It is our job as the pharmacist to protect the safety of the patient. But sometimes mistakes are still made. Sometimes physicians don't know the dosage of a medication. Sometimes we end up arguing with the doctor's secretary. I won't fill the prescription unless I talk to the doctor."

ARIAN MOINI, PHARMD, LOS ANGELES, CA

According to the Institute of Medicine, medication errors injure 1.5 million people a year. Unfortunately, medication errors can happen to anyone. From prescribing to filling your prescription, any medical professional involved can make a mistake.

The good news is, you can prevent it.

The most comprehensive and foolproof way to prevent medication mistakes is to take charge of the medications you currently take. Know their brand and generic names, dosages, which medical condition you are taking each for and what each medicine looks like.

"A prescription was called in for 500mg of Keflex and 250mg Zantac. We (pharmacy) typed it and filled it correctly. The patient's husband came in to pick up his wife's prescription late afternoon. An ancillary staff member handed him another

patient's medication by mistake, a patient's name with a similar spelling. The other person's medication was a blood pressure medication. The patient took two doses of the wrong medication that night. She came in the next day and said, 'You gave me the wrong medication. This is for someone else.' I took her blood pressure. It was fine. I called her doctor and explained the incident. I sent the patient to his office. She was fine. But our clerk was so upset that he quit."

Anonymous PharmD, Chicago, IL

How Medication Errors Happen

- The doctor makes an error in transcription. This can surface in the form of a misspelling of the patient's name or the name of a medication.

- Illegible handwriting. Yes, it still happens. For example, a doctor writes out a prescription and the pharmacy misreads it or can't read it at all.

- The medical office emails or faxes a prescription to the pharmacy with writing that isn't clear. The quality of the scanned prescription or fax can be so poor that the pharmacist can't easily read it.

- The doctor calls in a prescription to the pharmacy. Because she's in a hurry, she talks quickly, which forces the pharmacist to write quickly. If a pharmacy technician fills that prescription, she may not interpret the pharmacist's handwriting correctly.

- The pharmacy tech interprets the prescription incorrectly.

- The patient has not provided a doctor with the names of all of the medications she is currently taking. For example: You see a specialist, such as a cardiologist. The doctor does not know you are taking Lopressor and gives you a prescription for the generic form

"Kapidex is similar to Casodex. When you have long hours and the pharmacist is multi-tasking, mistakes can be made. The prescription comes over the phone from the doctor's office. It can come from the secretary and not even the nurse. Mistakes can happen with everyone involved."

Arian Moini, PharmD, Los Angeles, CA

of Lopressor called metoprolol. You could end up taking double the dose of medication. Pay attention.

- The patient uses several pharmacies to fill her prescriptions. This puts each pharmacy in a position of not having complete information.

How to Prevent Medication Errors

Preventing medication mistakes is one the easiest and most successful tasks you can do. It is within your control.

> "No medication error is ever intentional."
>
> Peter Naysan, Pharm D,
> Los Angeles, CA

Create a List of All Your Medications

List all of your medications (include the generic and brand names of each), their dosages, and what medical condition you take them for. List allergies to medications. List over-the-counter medications, herbs and supplements. Some people think that anything sold over the counter is not medication. It is!

Some doctors insist that patients bring along all of their medication bottles to their appointments. Ask your doctor if you should do this.

Even if you go to an urgent care center or the ER, you must provide a list of your current medications.

You can keep this list on your smartphone, electronic tablet or on a piece of paper in your wallet or purse. Each time you see a doctor or other medical professional, you will present this list.

> "In the course of a day, about twenty percent of all prescriptions contain certain irregularities and questionable issues that need to be corrected in order to fill the prescription correctly. For example, bad handwriting renders the script undecipherable, errors with dosage might not match the drug, or the directions might not be appropriate."
>
> Peter Naysan, PharmD,
> Los Angeles, CA

In Chapter 3, I suggest creating a medical ID card to fit into one of the slots in your wallet. Mine is typed out on a folded piece of paper and is in the slot next to my driver's license. Among other information, my medical ID card includes a list of my current medications, their dosages and allergies to medications.

If you don't know what medications you are taking, their dosages, or what they are for, start by calling your doctor's office and asking questions. You can also call your pharmacist.

If You Receive a Prescription from Your Doctor

When you receive a new medication, ask your doctor the following questions:

- What is the name of the medication you prescribed for me? (Ask for both brand and generic names.)

- What is the dosage and how many times a day do I need to take it?

- Why am I taking this medication?

- Do I need to take this medication with or without food or at any particular time of day?

- Are there any side effects associated with this medication?

- How long do you want me to take this medication?

- Can this medication interact with any of my other medications?

Write down the answers in your medical journal. You may want to refer to them later.

Read Your New Prescription

So, you've gotten a new prescription from your doctor and it's in your pocket. Take it out and read it before you leave the doctor's office. If you are at all confused, ask the doctor for clarification before you walk out the door.

- Check your name on the prescription.

- Is the medication the same as what the doctor told you to take?

- Is the prescription possibly for a generic of the brand medication?

- Are dosing instructions the same as what the doctor told you?

- Ask questions before you leave your physician's office.

Filling Your New Prescription

Before you go to the pharmacy and hand over your prescription, know what the medication is, the dosage, and what medical condition it is for. Check to see that the prescription is what the doctor said it was in the office.

If not, call the doctor. If you need the medication urgently, page the doctor and explain the situation.

Several pharmacists reported the same story—that patients come from doctors' offices with prescriptions and they have no idea what the medications are and what they are for. They also said that many patients don't know their diagnoses.

> "Patients can prevent medication errors by writing down the name of their medication and directions for use. Patients should learn the names of their medicines."
>
> Molly Griffin, MD, Dermatology, Santa Monica, CA

If a pharmacist cannot read the prescription or she detects errors, she will call or page the doctor to try to rectify the problem. But according to some pharmacists, some doctors don't always call back.

One pharmacist who fills prescriptions for a major teaching hospital said, "Patients will come from seeing doctors at a teaching hospital. If there is a problem with the medication, as in a misspelling of the name of the medication or an incorrect dosage, we need to be able to call the doctor. Some patients don't know their doctors' names."

If you see a doctor, whether in a busy clinic or hospital, you must know who prescribed the medication for you. Write down the information before you leave the medical facility.

Know the answers to these questions:

- What is my doctor's name and contact information?

- What is the medication and dosage I have been given?

- What medical condition is it for?

- How often am I supposed to take it?

Pharmacists are trained to spot drug interactions and many have computer programs to catch medication errors and interactions but as a take-charge patient you must do your part. Why? Because you don't want to ingest a medication that you were not supposed to have.

Understand Why You Are Taking a Medication

Study after study shows that the more you understand about why you are taking your medicine, the more apt you are to take it as the doctor prescribed it. Ask questions.

Use Only One Pharmacy

You can do your part in preventing medication errors by using only one pharmacy. Each pharmacy keeps track of your medications in its computer and the computer is set up to alert the pharmacist if there is a drug interaction or possible medication allergy.

If your pharmacy or mail-order pharmacy has an auto refill program, consider participating in it for your medications that are repeatedly the same dose.

If you use more than one pharmacy, you must provide each pharmacy with a list of your current medications and dosages and allergies to medications. This will allow the pharmacies to prevent drug interactions.

Make an appointment ahead of time to see the pharmacist and go over all of your medications. This might be a little easier if you use an independent pharmacy. Remember to say thank you or express some form of gratitude. Pharmacists don't get paid extra to do this for you.

Consider Using an Independent Pharmacy

Independent pharmacies are recommended by many medical professionals because they tend to pay closer attention and can take more time to explain and answer medication questions.

Nothing against big chains, but you might find more personal attention at an independent pharmacy and might find it easier to develop a good working relationship with the pharmacist there.

Mail-Order Pharmacies

Mail-order pharmacies have cheap prices, but you may pay another price altogether.

Some potential problems:

- Patients have reported that they don't get their shipment of medications on time. Then they have to turn to their physicians to get extra medication to carry them through until the mail-order prescription arrives.

- Physicians can fax in prescription renewals and the pharmacy can lose the prescription.
- Patients have reported medication mix-ups with mail-order pharmacies.
- Mail-order pharmacies may not inform the patient that they are sending a new generic. The patient may receive a medication that is a different shape or color. The patient doesn't know if the medication was sent in error (wrong medication) or is a new generic.

If you do happen to receive a medication that doesn't look right, call your mail-order pharmacy and ask questions. However, if that is not successful, you might have to take the medication to your local pharmacy for advice.

Check Carefully If Your Doctor Called In, Emailed or Faxed the Prescription

There are times when your doctor will email or fax a prescription to the pharmacy. At these times it is even more important to know what medication you were prescribed and what it is for. Doctors' handwriting can be illegible. Office personnel who write, scan or type the prescription can make errors. Even faxing can muddy clarity of a prescription. The end result is that the pharmacist is left in the dark about what the medication is or how it should be given. This is the reason it is so important for you to know what you are being prescribed.

Check Your Medication When You Pick It Up from the Pharmacy

"A patient came in with a prescription for Keflex. I asked her about allergies to medications, in particular allergy to penicillin. She said that when she was a kid, her throat closed up on penicillin. She did not know her new prescription, Keflex, was related to penicillin. I advised her to not to take the medication and to call her doctor. She explained that she had just come from the emergency room at the hospital and no doctor had asked about medication allergies."

Arian Moini, PharmD, Los Angeles, CA

- When you pick up your prescription, read the label on the bottle to make sure you receive the correct prescription. Check your name on the bottle.

  There should be a label on the bottle that describes the color and shape of the pills. Open the bottle and check.

- When you receive a medication that you take regularly, make sure you recognize the pills. If you don't, do not take the pills until you have consulted with a pharmacist. Generics of the same medication can be produced by several different companies so your medicine might look different. Ask questions if your medication does not appear the same as the last time you received it.

- Before you leave the pharmacy, check to see that you have received the number of pills you were prescribed.

- Tell your pharmacist about any allergies to medications.

- Tell your pharmacist if you are breastfeeding or pregnant.

- You should receive a sheet of information about your medication when you pick it up. If you have a new medication, the pharmacist should give you a consult on your medicine. If not, you can request a medication consult with the pharmacist to go over any questions.

> "It is up to the patient to be proactive. Ask for instructions in your language."
>
> Arian Moini, PharmD,
> Los Angeles, CA

- You can ask if the pharmacy can translate the medication instructions in your language. Pharmacies don't have the ability to translate into many languages, but some are offered.

Use Your Pharmacist

Pharmacists are an untapped source for information for all patients. Several pharmacists said that patients come to them for further information about medications if they don't understand their doctors' explanations. One pharmacist explained that some patients feel more comfortable asking questions of a pharmacist outside a medical setting.

During my chronic pain condition, I consulted with two pharmacists about various medicines I was prescribed and each was very helpful. One caught a possible drug interaction with a prescription from a doctor who wasn't interested in seeing my list of current medications.

I talked to the other pharmacist about my chronic pain condition, and he connected me with a patient who was seeing a couple of the same physicians I was and who had symptoms very similar to mine. When I contacted her there was instant rapport, and we became good friends and supported each other as we sought solutions to our medical problems.

Get to Know Your Pharmacist

Go into your pharmacy and introduce yourself. Pharmacists are human beings just like us. You can establish a relationship with your pharmacist in the same way I have described establishing one with your doctor. Be friendly and respectful. You can share that you're new to her pharmacy and strike up a brief conversation.

You can then gauge if this pharmacist is a good match for you. Do you feel comfortable talking to her? Do you feel confident in her knowledge? If you were in need, would you feel comfortable calling this pharmacist? If the answer is no, find another pharmacist, even one in the same pharmacy.

You can always call and ask questions of the pharmacist about prescriptions or over-the-counter-medications.

Choose Good Times to Call Your Pharmacist

Several pharmacists said to avoid phone calls between 4 PM and 8 PM. That is when people get off work and have their prescriptions filled. Good times to call are early in the morning, between 12 PM and 1 PM when doctors' offices are closed, before 4 PM and after 8 PM.

Express Appreciation

If a pharmacist helps you with questions about medications, be sure you say thank you and show gratitude. Pharmacists don't get paid extra for their time spent with you. If you appreciate their time, it paves the way for a good relationship in the future. You want your pharmacist to remember you. If there is ever a time you are in need, a good relationship pays you back. So consider investing a small amount of time and energy in anticipation of a good relationship for the future.

Make an Appointment for a Consultation with Your Pharmacist

Consider meeting with your pharmacist if you take multiple medications. This will help you manage your medications and prevent errors. If you see several doctors who have prescribed medications, it is a good idea.

Call or stop by the pharmacy and ask the pharmacist when a good time would be to go over your medications. A big chain pharmacy may not have time to do this if they are in a busy metropolitan area but it doesn't hurt to ask.

Before Your Consultation:

Go over all your medications. Create a list of questions and write them down in your medical journal. Bring your medical journal with you so that you can write down the answers.

Sample questions:

- I'm confused about all the medications I'm taking. Can you please go over them with me?

- What is each medication for?

- Which are brand name and which are generic?

- Do any of my medications cause side effects? What are they?

- Are there alternatives to some of my medications that don't cause these side effects?

- I don't remember exactly when I'm supposed to take my medications. Can you give me guidance?

- Can you give me some ideas on how to keep track of my medications?

Maximize Your Relationship with Your Pharmacist

Most pharmacists said that they remember the really nice customers and the really nasty ones. Some claimed to go out of their way for a really nice customer.

> "I have my favorite patients. They become a priority. It's all in how you talk to the pharmacist."
>
> Soo Jin Shin, PharmD,
> Los Angeles, CA

What do you think pharmacists said about the nasty customers? They admitted to trying to stay out of their way. If you want good service and want to maximize your relationship with your pharmacist (yes, you do) then be nice, even if you experience a problem with the pharmacy. You can be firm and do everything in your power to correct the problem and still remain cordial. If you don't see an end to your problem with the pharmacy, find a new one. It's certainly worth your time.

Managing Your Medications

If you are taking multiple medications, here are some tips to manage and organize them.

- Ask your doctor for a once-a-day pill or a combination, such as a "fixed dose" combination. For example, Caduet is a combination of blood pressure and cholesterol medication.

- Ask your pharmacist for a "blister pack." Medications are placed in bubble cards and marked with the day, time of day and dose. There may be a nominal fee.

- Some doctors like their patients to keep all medications in their original bottles. Mark on the bottle in big letters what the medication is and what it is for (e.g., high blood pressure, diabetes, thyroid, etc.). Several doctors suggested bringing in all of your prescription bottles to office visits.

- Many doctors and pharmacists recommend seven-day organizers. These can be purchased at any pharmacy.

- Some specialty pharmacies will send out your medications in a seven-day organizer box if you are disabled, elderly or have a serious medical condition. Ask your pharmacy if they will do this for you. Be sure to ask if there is an extra fee for this.

- Some pharmacies will also send charts with descriptions of the medications and instructions on how to take them. Ask if your pharmacy can do this for you.

- Enlist the help of a good friend or family member to set up your medications for each week.

- Take a photo of each medication and mark the name and what it is for on the photo. Create a board with photos of the pills and bottles.

- Keep a calendar and mark each time you take a medication. List the name, dosage and time.

- Use a timer on your smartphone, electronic tablet, cell phone or watch to remind you to take your medication.

- If you have several pills to take each day while you are away from home, consider purchasing an organizer from your pharmacy. As an alternative, one pharmacist suggested using small baggies with a label for each pill type and the time it is to be taken.

How to Get Medication Refills When You Travel

If you plan to travel, the best thing to do is to get your prescriptions refilled before you leave and take all the medication you need with you. This is imperative if you are traveling outside of the United States.

If you get caught short in the United States, in most cases you can get refills if you have them.

If your prescriptions are with a big chain pharmacy such as CVS, your information is in the computer and your records will pop up at any CVS pharmacy.

If you have the option of keeping your prescriptions at a small local pharmacy, be sure you have their contact information with you. If you run out of medication, you can call and have them contact a pharmacy near you (you may have to find this pharmacy and obtain their contact information). This way you may be able to get at least enough medication to get you home.

Tips to Expedite Filling Prescriptions

- Ask your doctor's office to call in, fax, or email your prescription before you arrive at the pharmacy (make sure your doctor has your pharmacy's contact information).

- Call the pharmacy before you arrive and ask if they received the prescription from your doctor.

- Ask your pharmacy when your medicine will be ready.

- Know the name of your medication, the dosage and what it is for.

- Know the name of your diagnosis and have the doctor's phone number with you in case there are questions.

A Few Medication Safety Tips

- Know the expiration dates of your medicines.

- For liquid medication, such as for your children, be sure to use a premeasured syringe or spoon to get the accurate dosage. This means that the teaspoon you use for your coffee in the morning is not an accurate measurement. You can purchase a measurement spoon or syringe at your pharmacy.

- Many medical professionals suggested keeping a two-week supply of medication you take regularly on hand in the event of an emergency. If you are going to travel, you may need additional medication. Plan ahead.

I Ran Out of My Medication!

It's happened to all of us. It's a Friday afternoon at 4 o'clock and it's the start of a holiday weekend. Your thyroid medication is something you must take every day and this morning you took your last pill. Whoops!

At this point, all you can do is hope you have a refill on that prescription. If you do, call your pharmacy and speak to the pharmacist. Ask if she can fill the prescription by the end of the day. If the answer is yes, when you go to pick up your prescription, express appreciation to the pharmacist.

"I see patients with asthma. Some are passive about it. A few let their medications expire and then they come in with a respiratory illness with a really bad asthma exacerbation. Pay attention!"

Darlene Petersen, MD,
Family Medicine, Roy, UT

If you do not have a refill on that prescription, call your doctor's office right away. Hopefully, you can get a refill. If not, you might have to page the doctor. If this happens, you will have to apologize because this is your error and as a take-charge patient you try not to do this.

If you cannot get through to the doctor, ask your pharmacist if she can give you enough medication to get you through the weekend.

When Do I Take My Medication Again?

A few pharmacists and doctors suggested managing your medications on your smartphone, electronic tablet or other device. You might have to get a special application, but you can set timers on your phone to alert you to take a certain medication.

You can also keep a list of your medications on your phone so that when you need it, it's right there.

I'm Going to Stop This Medication!

"I have a patient, a woman in her late seventies. She was very vibrant, spunky. She never saw doctors. She came to see me because she needed cataract surgery done. The eye doctor would not do the surgery because her blood pressure was so high. I gave her blood pressure medication. She got the surgery. She came back because of an illness. Her blood pressure was higher than when I had first seen her. She'd stopped the medication because she didn't want to be on medications. Now she's had a stroke and is in a nursing home.

It's just sad. Why didn't she at least meet with me to discuss why she wanted to stop the blood pressure medication? I could have discussed options, alternatives."

Linda Nadwodny, DO, FAAFP, Family Medicine, Lansdale, PA

"The fact that your medication is not working may suggest that the initial diagnosis wasn't correct. Disorders present in different stages and with different symptoms in different people. The doctor was not 'wrong' in beginning treatment for what it looked like at the time. If you don't go back for re-evaluation, then the doctor won't know."

Anonymous MD, Santa Monica, CA

Every doctor was emphatic about patients not stopping their medications because they think they are not working or because the side effects are unacceptable. Get in touch with your doctor. Let her know what you are experiencing with your medication. There may be alternatives, or you may simply need to be reassured that your particular medication takes time to work.

Medication Side Effects

If you start a new medication and begin to have new symptoms, talk to your doctor. Describe the new symptoms you are experiencing.

> *"I have an older patient. She came in and said, it's so hard to exercise. My legs ache so much. I looked at her medication list. I asked her, 'How long have you been on Lipitor? Did you tell your doctor?'"*
>
> Anonymous MD, Philadelphia, PA

If you develop new symptoms, try researching the new medication on the internet (using only credible websites) or call your pharmacist to find out if there might be a correlation.

Often, side effects wear off with time. Discuss this with your doctor and your pharmacist.

Remember, you know your body best.

Drug Interactions

Each time you see a doctor who gives you a prescription for a new medication, be sure that doctor has a list of your current medications and dosages.

You can also ask your pharmacist to look up your medications and make sure there aren't any interactions with the medications you are currently taking. You might think, "I don't need to do that. My doctor wouldn't give me a medication that would interact with other medications I am taking."

Think again.

Your doctor wouldn't give you a medication that would cause a drug interaction if she were aware of it. How many specialists do you see? Does every single one have a list of your current medications and dosages? Probably not, unless you have provided it.

> "If you take a variety of sleep medications, be careful. If you combine medications, be careful. Your doctor may give you a sleep medication, and he/she may not know that you are taking alcohol on top of it. People inadvertently do damage to themselves. For example: a patient has problems falling asleep and he takes a pill to sleep. He still cannot sleep and takes a narcotic medication to help him relax and sleep on top of the previous pill. If he is also taking an anti-seizure medication, these medicines are at least additive in terms of causing the inability to breathe normally and deeply while asleep."
>
> Joseph J. Morgan, MD, President, Pharmaceutical Industry Consultants, Yardley, PA

"Ask your pharmacist about any possible drug interactions with your medications. If you have impairment of the liver or kidneys, stay on top of this. Some drugs will affect one or the other system since most drugs are metabolized via the kidneys or liver, some interact specifically with each other, and all drugs have side effects worth knowing about. For example, if you go to an orthopedist for knee pain, you may receive a new prescription for a medication that could interact with another and all because this doctor doesn't know what you are taking or potentially what interactions the drugs you are taking have."

Joseph J. Morgan, MD, President,
Pharmaceutical Industry Consultants, Yardley, PA

Important Information about Medications

Generics

What is a generic drug? The FDA considers a generic drug to be identical or bioequivalent to a brand name drug in dosage form, safety, strength, route of administration, and quality. *Bioequivalent* means only that the "active" ingredients need to be the same. According to two pharmacists, when it comes to generic equivalency to brand medication, the FDA allows for 10 percent plus or minus of the content of the drug.

Generic drugs are cheaper than brand-name drugs. Not all brand-name drugs have generics.

Generics Can Be Confusing

Once a drug is available generically, many different companies will make it. This means that generics can come in all shapes, colors and sizes. Confusion can occur at this point. This is when you must call your pharmacist and ask questions or bring in the generic if you don't recognize it and ask the pharmacist questions.

If your doctor prescribes a brand-name medication for you for which a generic is available, your insurance company may choose to reimburse you only for the cost of the generic medication. Be sure to ask questions about the generic you have been prescribed and go over the list of medications you are already taking. Many doctors told stories about patients receiving a brand medication from one doctor and the generic of the same medication from another doctor, and the patients didn't know they were the same drug.

As a result they had doubled the dose. Ask questions!

Most physicians think that generics are great. A few said to beware if you order them yourself on the internet without a prescription.

> "Generics can be very confusing. If we only have brand name medications, it would be less confusing. Most brand name medications have the name on the pill and there is only one pill on the market."
>
> Soo Jin Shin, PharmD, Los Angeles, CA

What If the Pills You Receive Are Different Shapes and Colors

It is possible that you will get a generic of one shape and color one month and the same generic in a different shape and color (from a different pharmaceutical company) the next month.

If this is confusing, call your pharmacist and ask questions. You can say something like, "I received my prescription for x medication today. The shape/color are different than the pills I received last month. Would you mind checking? I just want to make sure I have the correct medication. Thank you."

Drug Advertising in the Media

Drug companies use all forms of media to sell their medications directly to patients. As a take-charge patient you need to understand that the symptoms they list in advertisements may not apply to you and that it is the drug company's goal to encourage you to ask for their medications from your doctor.

> "Don't fall victim to drug advertising. Do your own thinking as a patient. Be able to discriminate what is just advertising, especially by the drug companies."
>
> Rafael Reisfeld, MD, General Surgery, Los Angeles, CA

Use credible websites to do your own research on medications. Talk to your doctor about what might be appropriate for you.

PATIENT SAFETY CHECKLIST

- ☐ Do I know the name and dosage of the medication my doctor prescribed?

- ☐ Do I understand why I am taking this medication?

- ☐ Do I understand how to take this medication?

- ☐ Do I know the brand and generic names of this medication?

- ☐ Did I review the prescription in the doctor's office?

- ☐ Did I look at the medication at the pharmacy?

- ☐ Do I need to set up an appointment to meet with my pharmacist?

- ☐ Do I need help managing my medications?

- ☐ Have I explored my options to get help to manage my medications?

- ☐ Have I created a list of all my medications?

- ☐ Have I considered using only one pharmacy?

- ☐ Do I need to set up timers to alert me to take my medications?

12

How to Manage Medical Errors
Misdiagnosis, Missed Diagnosis and No Diagnosis

*"The astute physician knows when to say, 'I do not
know' and when to ask for another opinion.
Keeping an open mind to any and all possibilities
will more than likely yield the correct diagnosis and
treatment. It is when we make quick, formulated
decisions that we fall into the misdiagnosis abyss."*

JACK C. ROSENFELD, MD,
FAMILY MEDICINE AND GERIATRICS, LANSDALE, PA

M edical errors are preventable errors, whether or not they are harmful to the patient. They can include inaccurate or incomplete diagnoses of diseases, injuries or medical conditions. Medical errors also occur when medical professionals make correct diagnoses but choose incorrect treatments. Medical errors occur in hospitals, clinics, surgery centers, doctors' offices, nursing homes, pharmacies, and patients' homes. They can involve medicines, surgeries, diagnoses, equipment or lab reports. Patient safety is a team effort. Be an active member of your health care team!

Medical errors can occur in or with

- medicines,
- diagnoses,
- surgeries,

- procedures,
- test results,
- lab reports,
- equipment.

Misdiagnosis

According to Peter Pronovost, MD, a patient-safety researcher at Johns Hopkins University, misdiagnoses (diagnostic errors) kill 40,000 to 80,000 hospitalized patients annually. They are the leading cause of malpractice suits.

> "Being a good diagnostician is like a being great detective."
>
> Jack C. Rosenfeld, MD, Family Medicine and Geriatrics, Lansdale, PA

A misdiagnosis occurs when a medical professional inaccurately comes to a conclusion about what is wrong with the patient. About one in twenty inpatient hospital deaths is attributed to misdiagnosed illnesses. Inside or outside of the hospital, about one in six of us, throughout our lifetime, will be subjected to a misdiagnosis by a medical professional.

Doctors are not the only medical professionals who misdiagnose. Consider the pathologists and radiologists who read your tests. One doctor told me that he always looks at his patients' MRIs with the radiologist because radiologists can make mistakes too. He recently caught a hairline fracture in a patient's MRI that the radiologist had deemed "unremarkable."

Remember, you can always ask that a test be reread or redone if you have doubts about the diagnosis.

During my sixteen months of chronic pain, I received ten misdiagnoses from eleven physicians. It is shocking to me even now that I went through this. It was not clear to me at the time of each misdiagnosis that it was in fact incorrect. Three specialists rejected my first misdiagnosis of interstitial cystitis (IC), so I knew that was wrong. But with the rest of the misdiagnoses, because most came from very respected physicians, some affiliated with highly respected medical schools, I honestly wasn't sure until I had undergone medical treatments and procedures that didn't work. I gave most doctors I saw a fair chance. Unless there is a warning sign or clear sign of a misdiagnosis, how are we as patients to know until we've tried treatment plans that fail?

Most of the misdiagnoses I received contradicted all the others. Perhaps this was partly due to the specialties of the physicians I saw and also partly due to the fact that hernias in women are pretty rare. Who knew? None of the eleven doctors did. Perhaps they didn't consider hernias as a possibility because hernias are outside of their specialties. As I've said before, specialists can focus on the part of the body they specialize in and neglect other possibilities.

I know that if I had not become a take-charge patient, with all that entails, and kept pursuing answers, I would still be in chronic pain. My persistence and research led me to Dr. T., who diagnosed me correctly and cured me. One key component to this success story is that I trusted my instincts when I read the article about hernias in women (see Chapter 1). When I read about the woman described in that article who had the same symptoms and profile I did, I felt in my gut that I had the same diagnosis. If I had not trusted my instincts and pursued the doctor in that article, I know I would still be where I was—in debilitating pain, discouraged and worn down. I am now pain free and have gotten my life back.

If you are going through something similar and have not yet received an accurate diagnosis, embrace the concepts of a take-charge patient that I've outlined in this book. Continue with your search for an accurate diagnosis. Don't give up. Keep pursuing answers. Do your research. Gather support for yourself. It may not be easy, but if you don't give up, you will find an accurate diagnosis and treatment plan like I did.

> *"I went to see my ophthalmologist for my annual check-up at which time I was told that I should schedule a cataract lens replacement. I was contacted by their "lens expert" who did an up-sell to an "accommodating intraocular lens" which allows the eye to focus much as it does with normal vision. Unfortunately, these lenses are not covered by insurance so it would have been an out-of-pocket expense paid to the ophthalmologist.*
>
> *I did some research on the surgery and decided to get a second opinion from another ophthalmologist who examined*

me and did a corneal mapping which the other ophthalmologist never did. It was determined that I did not in fact have cataracts but a condition called keratoconus, a non-treatable, degenerative condition of the cornea that has nothing to do with cataracts. Surgery was not recommended by the new ophthalmologist as it wouldn't have helped my condition. I had the second opinion confirmed by an expert in my condition at Cedars-Sinai Medical Center, Los Angeles.

I had a high level of trust and confidence in my first ophthalmologist as I had been his patient for over 20 years. I was troubled by the misdiagnosis and being told to simply 'have the surgery.' Had I done so, my vision would have been permanently impaired by an unnecessary surgery."

Bruce, Patient, Van Nuys, CA

Why Misdiagnoses Occur

There are several reasons misdiagnoses can occur. They include the following:

- "Premature closure"—a failure on the part of the medical professional to consider all possible diagnoses. Doctors are taught in medical school to go with the most common diagnoses first and can miss considering rare or uncommon diagnoses.

- Specialists who see only their specialty instead of the patient's whole body.

- Lab tests that are not ordered or test results that are not followed up on.

- Patients who see several different health care providers who do not communicate with one another.

- Patients who do not provide a complete health summary and history.

- Poor communication between doctors and their patients.

Tips to Help Prevent Misdiagnoses

- Come prepared to the doctor visit with copies of pertinent medical records, and your health summary, which incluces a list of medications and their dosages, over-the-counter medications, herbs and supplements, allergies to medications and more. (See Chapter 3 for more information.) Be prepared to present a packet of information to each and every doctor you see. This also prevents the problem of misplaced, lost or inaccurate medical records.

- Come prepared with a list of questions.

- Ask for a diagnosis from your doctor. Ask why it is suspected.

- Ask your doctor if there are any other possible diagnoses for what you have.

- Enlist a family member or good friend to be your advocate. She will be your second set of eyes and ears. Ask her to take notes on conversations with physicians, whether you are in a doctor's office or in the hospital.

- Create a list of all your symptoms. If you are in the hospital, ask your advocate to help you with this. Record the time of day your symptoms occur and what makes them better or worse. List what you have tried to make the symptoms better.

- Follow up on your test results. If you are in the hospital or seeing a medical professional in an office, ask for your test results and for a copy of them.

- Research your condition or diagnostic tests online or at your local library. If you are in the hospital, ask your advocate to do this for you. Your hospital may have a library with information.

- Research your diagnosis. If you are uncertain about it, create a list of questions and make a time to talk to your doctor.

- Get a second opinion. If you are unconvinced about the diagnosis you are given or simply are not getting better, find another doctor to give you a second opinion, preferably one who is board certified in her specialty and who is affiliated with a respected medical school.

- Ask for lab tests to be repeated. Doctors can make mistakes, as can radiologists, pathologists or lab technicians.

Speak up. Ask questions. Be assertive. Many of us are nervous or anxious when talking with our doctors or other medical professionals. Remember that you know your body best, and the more information you gather and contribute, the more confident you will feel.

Remember that your body never lies to you. Take it seriously.

A year ago, I injured the little toe on my right foot. The toe stuck out like a chicken wing. My internist saw me at the end of the day and diagnosed it as fractured and dislocated. Because he didn't have an x-ray machine that could accommodate a foot, he suggested that I go to the ER, since fixing the dislocation might be easier before swelling set in.

Four hours into my ER visit, the ER doctor read my x-rays and said that my toe was not dislocated but only fractured. Based on my internist's evaluation and my own instincts, I felt that diagnosis was incorrect. The ER nurse proceeded to try to force my toe into place so that she could tape it to the adjoining toe. The pain was excruciating. I asked her to stop, but she persisted. Finally I stated firmly that I was leaving the hospital with my x-rays. The next morning my podiatrist read the same x-rays and said that my toe was indeed dislocated and badly fractured. He explained that he would have to do a procedure to repair it.

This experience made me realize the importance of listening to my own instincts even in the face of opposition from medical professionals.

Missed Diagnosis or No Diagnosis

Sometimes a diagnosis can be missed simply because the symptoms have not progressed far enough for a physician to be able to make an accurate diagnosis. A diagnosis can be missed because the medical professional didn't consider other possible diagnoses, the doctor was not given enough information from the patient, the doctor was rushed or tests results were inaccurate.

Keep pursuing answers. Trust your instincts. You know your body better than anyone.

"I went to my internist with a horrible sore throat. I had been taking 150mg of Zantac a day for acid reflux as prescribed by him. My internist diagnosed me with an upper respiratory infection and

gave me the antibiotic, Amoxicillin. When my condition didn't improve, I went back to see my internist. This time the doctor gave me a prescription for another round of antibiotics plus a prescription steroid inhaler. After taking this medication and using the inhaler as directed, my sore throat became much worse. I could hardly swallow. My wife urged me to see an ear nose and throat doctor whom she knew. This ENT doctor was not part of my health plan but my wife urged me to pay out of pocket. I saw the new doctor. He took one look at my throat and asked, "Are you being treated for acid reflux?" I said yes, that I was taking Zantac 150mg per day as prescribed by my internist.

This new ENT doctor said that my throat condition was a direct result of acid coming up and burning my throat and was not a result of a respiratory infection. He said the antibiotics I was on were not the correct treatment for my condition and that the steroid inhaler made the condition worse. He put me on Nexium. My throat got dramatically better in a few days."

Henry, Patient, North Hampton, MA

"If a patient's team of doctors is unable to diagnose a patient or if his/her doctors all disagree on either a diagnosis or treatment plan, the patient should be proactive and go to a teaching hospital with a renowned reputation. If the patient has a terminal disease or one that has no proven treatments, the patient may opt to join an experimental clinical trial study."

Fran Ginsberg, Medical Office Manager, Santa Monica, CA

"Know your family history. It may be key to identifying difficult-to-diagnose conditions."

H. Kenneth Schueler, Professional Patient Advocate, New York, NY

Tips to Help If You Have a Missed Diagnosis or No Diagnosis

- Enlist support for yourself.

- Become your own medical detective. Start doing research using credible websites. Join online support groups and share information.

- Meet with your PCP and ask her what she thinks your diagnosis could be, which tests might reveal the problem, which specialists she thinks you might see and where to get more information.

- Find a doctor who is affiliated with a highly respected medical institution and who specializes in what you think you might have. Make an appointment for a consultation and ask questions. Bring copies of all your pertinent medical records.

   Once this doctor has reviewed your records, ask what she thinks your diagnosis could be, where she thinks you can go for help, and whether there is anyone she knows who may be of help to you.

- Go to the National Institutes of Health, Undiagnosed Diseases Program website at http://rarediseases.info.nih.gov/.aspx?PageID=31.

The diagnosis journey is no fun. I did it for over a year before I found a doctor who finally gave me an accurate diagnosis and treatment plan. It was not easy. Be persistent and don't give up. Keep researching, enlist loved ones to research as well and discuss your findings together. Get more opinions from doctors. The more knowledge you have, the more empowered you will feel. Become an expert on your symptoms and on what you and your doctors suspect you may have.

If you can, hire a professional patient advocate to help you with your diagnosis journey.

If you have a family member or good friend who is a physician, reach out for help. Ask for direction.

"I had a patient, a thirty-eight year old man. He had pain in his arms. He went to see three neurologists and didn't get any results. He started having reactions to medications the doctors gave him. As with any patient in his situation, he felt like he was given a "garbage can diagnosis" which is a description of symptoms when we don't really know the cause. He was terrified. He got seven, eight, and nine opinions, all from top people at UCLA, Mayo Clinic, etc. All the opinions contradicted each other. The patient, in this case, had to be very proactive with research and was eventually able to partially eliminate his symptoms."

Roger E. Dafter, PhD, Associate Director,
Mind-Body Medicine Group, Division of Head and Neck Surgery,
UCLA David Geffen School of Medicine, Los Angeles, CA

Could Your Problem Be Side Effects from a New Medication?

If you develop new symptoms after starting a new medication, consider the possibility that this new medication could be causing your symptoms.

Many of us don't think of medication as a possible cause of symptoms, but many have side effects that aren't listed in the information that accompanies them.

If you have new symptoms and you have recently started taking a new medication, call your doctor and ask questions. You can also research the medication online, at your local library or ask questions of your pharmacist. If your symptoms don't match the side-effect profile of the new medication you are taking, it may have nothing to do with it, but consider the following story:

> "A patient always has to be on their toes. When a new symptom occurs, you should immediately try to research a medication you are on and also research drug interactions. This should be the patient's first line of defense."
>
> Fran Ginsberg, Medical Office Manager, Santa Monica, CA

> "When I was in my early forties, I went to a urologist because I suddenly started having bladder spasms and difficulty urinating. Upon examination, my prostate was not enlarged. I informed the urologist I was taking (a popular allergy/decongestant medication) for my allergies. The urologist never suggested that a medication I was taking could have been the cause of my symptoms. This urologist put me through painful biopsies, expensive scans, and put me on a prostate medication for my symptoms.
>
> My wife did her own research on the internet and read that (a popular allergy/decongestant medicine) can cause prostate symptoms. As soon as I discontinued taking it my symptoms disappeared.
>
> I lost so much time from work, spent a lot of money, suffered through pain and took a prostate medication I did not need—all because of a misdiagnosis."
>
> Anonymous Patient, Miami, FL

Drug side effects or interactions may be responsible for new symptoms. A patient can also take medication for many years and then suddenly develop a reaction to it.

Be Persistent

If you are still experiencing symptoms and have yet to get an accurate diagnosis from a doctor, keep pursuing answers. You know your body, and if you have received diagnoses that don't seem correct, you must trust yourself and keep pursuing other medical opinions. If the medical treatment you are undertaking is not helping you to get better, get tough and keep looking.

If you have *no* diagnosis, don't let that stop you. You must persist even if you are caught up in the diagnosis journey.

Press on. Your body doesn't lie. Don't give up hope. You will find a diagnosis. Sometimes it just takes time and finding the correct set of eyes and ears.

Get Second, Third and Fourth Opinions

Find a board-certified physician who is affiliated with a respected medical institution and specializes in the area of your body where you experience the most symptoms. Schedule a consultation. Bring copies of your pertinent medical records and health summary with you.

Enlist Support from Your Loved Ones

For those who are on the diagnosis journey, you know it can be rough. It was for me. I relied on my husband and good friends to support me and spur me on. I discussed my symptoms with my husband and a couple of medically savvy friends. We all came up with ideas.

> "My twenty-nine-year-old boyfriend had severe bloating, constipation and stomach pain. He was an HMO patient. He went to see his primary care physician at the HMO facility. He was told he had irritable bowel syndrome and was advised to eat a high fiber diet. His doctor also said his stomach pain was probably stress related.
>
> After a few months, I took him to the emergency room at his HMO facility. He couldn't button his pants, despite the fact that he had lost weight. His stomach pain was becoming increasingly

unmanageable and severe. He was still very constipated and went days without moving his bowels. The emergency room doctor ordered a stomach x-ray and told him he was impacted. He was given an enema. He was also given a sigmoidoscopy that was negative. He was told to come back in a few weeks for follow-up and more testing. The doctor said he probably had diverticulitis based on his family history.

My boyfriend called for an appointment with his primary doctor the day after his emergency room visit. He was told they didn't have any openings for three weeks. He pleaded for an earlier appointment but was told there were no openings. Three weeks later he was given a barium enema and the results were negative. His primary care doctor told him he must have had a one-time episode and that he was fine.

He came home and told me he couldn't understand why he wasn't being taken seriously. He never went to doctors unless he had an acute problem. He became disillusioned with doctors. He started doubting himself and thought maybe he had a psychosomatic illness.

After nine months, he could no longer work or function. His stomach was distended and the pain was now unbearable. I took him to the emergency room at the HMO facility. Once again, the ER doctor didn't think he had a serious condition. I became upset and demanded that his doctor refer him to a gastroenterologist immediately. Being the daughter of a doctor, I knew this kind of treatment was unacceptable.

After waiting two weeks for an appointment, I took him to see a gastroenterologist. I told this doctor that my boyfriend's condition had been going on for one year. I explained that my father was a doctor and that he felt a colonoscopy was the next step. Luckily, this doctor took us seriously and scheduled a colonoscopy.

My boyfriend waited ten days to have a colonoscopy. The colonoscopy revealed metastatic cancer which had spread throughout his entire abdomen. He was told that he would have *to wait three weeks for surgery. My father, a physician, called the HMO and spoke to the gastroenterologist and begged her to expedite the surgery date. My boyfriend was operated on four days later. He had to go through extensive chemotherapy after he recovered from surgery."*

Anonymous Friend of the Patient, Los Angeles, CA

Find Support Groups

Members of support groups who have the same medical condition and/or disease tend to share research, names of good doctors who have helped them, emotional support and much more.

PATIENT SAFETY CHECKLIST

☐ Am I prepared for each doctor with copies of pertinent medical records, health summary, list of medications, list of symptoms, etc.?

☐ Do I have a list of questions?

☐ Did I research my diagnosis?

☐ Did I ask my doctor if there could be other possible diagnoses?

☐ Do I know my family history?

☐ Do I need to get a second opinion?

☐ Did I follow up on my test results?

☐ Did I ask what my test results mean?

☐ Did I ask for my tests to be repeated?

☐ Do I need to find a doctor affiliated with a highly respected medical school?

☐ Have I enlisted support from loved ones?

☐ Do I need an advocate?

13

How to Research Your Medical Conditions, Medications and Treatments

"The more knowledge a patient has about their medical condition, the more the patient will be empowered in making decisions concerning their care. This is the basis for a successful patient/physician partnership."

H. KENNETH SCHUELER,
PROFESSIONAL PATIENT ADVOCATE, NEW YORK, NY

As tempting as it may be, take-charge patients do not simply "Google" their symptoms, medical condition or illness. We have so much information at our fingertips that it is tempting to simply plug in search terms and go from there. However, you will not find credible information this way and in all likelihood you will find scary testimonials that may not be grounded in fact.

Anyone can set up a website and put health and medical information on the internet. Any of it may look credible, but as a take-charge patient, you know that you must be discerning about where you look on the internet. This is extremely important when you do research on your health, medical condition and treatment.

Which Are Credible Websites?

Go to academic, government and professional medical society/academy websites for the most credible information.

Look for websites that end in .gov, .org or .edu. If you do research using any of the websites listed in the Resources section of this book, you can comfortably share this information with your doctor and not lose credibility in her eyes. If you bring in information from a website or blog that is not respected, your doctor may not take your research seriously.

Here are some examples of respected websites:

- Centers for Disease Control and Prevention
  http://www.cdc.gov

- Memorial Sloan-Kettering Cancer Center
  http://www.mskcc.org

- American Cancer Society
  http://www.cancer.org

- Harvard Medical School
  http://hms.harvard.edu/hms/home.asp

Many doctors expressed frustration about patients bringing in information that was not credible and how much time they had to spend discrediting it. This is a waste of time for you and your doctor.

> *"I have a patient who is post-menopausal. She had upper abdominal pain. She went to a website, put in one symptom 'Abdominal pain' and came in for an ultrasound because she was worried about ovarian cancer. She had picked one disease from the long list and ignored the other symptoms for ovarian cancer, which she didn't have. With a few questions about the type of pain, we found it was exactly the same as when she had been previously treated for acid reflux. 'Googling' isolated symptoms causes a lot of anxiety. It can also cost the patient if they insist on tests to rule out serious but unlikely conditions based on one symptom of a long list."*
>
> Susan Tritt, MD, FACOG, Obstetrics and Gynecology,
> Santa Monica, CA

How to Do Research

If you do research before you have seen your doctor, keep in mind that many symptoms can have many causes. If you can hold off, wait until you see your doctor. Ask her for information and websites she likes and then do your own research.

Believe me, I've done my share of internet research even on credible websites and scared myself because my symptoms came up with scary diagnoses.

Be careful not to diagnose yourself before you see the doctor. You are not the expert—she is.

> *"I had a young girl comes to see me. She says, 'I think I'm hypothyroid. I'm tired.' I draw her blood. Thyroid is not the problem. She insists it is and tells me that she researched it on the internet. I had to go over her history. She insisted she could get thyroid meds on the internet."*
>
> Jo Ann C. Pullen, MD, Internal Medicine and Geriatrics,
> Los Angeles, CA

If you bring in research, most doctors will appreciate that you are taking an active interest in your health or medical condition. But many doctors dread patients who come in with fringe information from websites that are not credible or with extraneous information from their mother, aunt or friend.

Look for Repeating Information

When you find at least three credible websites, see if you find repeating information on them. This means that the three websites offer about the same information concerning your illness, medical condition, medication or treatment plan. This will give you a good idea of what is commonly accepted regarding your condition.

Ask for Handouts

Ask your doctor to give you handouts with information on your medical issue. If she does not have what you need, ask where you can find more information. Explain that you feel better knowing as much as you can so you can participate in your medical care.

Consider Second Opinions

Part of doing effective research is getting a second or third opinion on your diagnosis and/or treatment plan.

After you have researched the doctor you wish to see for a second opinion, make an appointment for a consultation. You will have to bring in copies of medical records pertaining to your medical issue, recent test results, recent reports from other doctors, your health summary and medical journal.

Create a list of questions for this doctor ahead of time and write down her answers to your questions in your medical journal.

Use Public Libraries

Our public librarians are trained to help people do research. If you want more information about an illness, medical condition, test or treatment plan, ask a librarian for help. She should be able to point out resources for you.

Read Health and Medical Blogs

Consider turning to health and medical blogs as part of your research process. Be discerning about which blogs you read, as anyone can start a blog and it may or may not be credible.

Start with a doctor's, nurse's or pharmacist's blog. I like KevinMD.com.

You can use health and medical blogs to learn about your diagnosis, symptoms, treatment plans, resources, doctors and other medical professionals. Discuss information you've uncovered with your doctor.

Join Online Groups and Forums

Through Facebook, Twitter, LinkedIn, chat rooms and online support groups, you can find others who either share your medical condition or are caring for those who do. You can find information on your medical condition from other patients in online groups and forums. You'll find out which treatment plans they have found helpful, which doctors they like and more. Other patients can be a wonderful source of information and can provide support for you.

How to Find Online Groups and Forums

Several doctors suggested simply using Google and searching for "support group" and your particular disease. For example, "breast cancer support groups." A number of groups will pop up. You can also ask your doctor for good online support groups.

Another good option is to go to a website for a particular disease or medical condition (for example: the American Cancer Society or the American Diabetes Association) and see if they have online support groups. If there is no mention on the website, call the number on the website or email the question to them.

Email Your Contacts

If you need medical information, consider casting a wide net.

One take-charge patient suggested emailing everyone in your email address book. She reported that when her son was diagnosed with a rare tumor, she emailed all of her business, friend and family contacts and asked if anyone had information on the type of tumor her son had and if anyone knew of specialists who could be helpful. Her brother-in-law received the email and forwarded it to his doctor. The brother-in-law emailed her back and said his doctor recommended a renowned doctor at Johns Hopkins in Baltimore, Maryland.

You never know who will help you.

PATIENT CHECKLIST

☐ Do I know which are credible websites for my research?

☐ Did I see my doctor first before I did research?

☐ Did I ask my doctor for handouts and websites for my research?

☐ Did I find the same information from more than two sources of information?

☐ Did I discuss my research findings with my doctor?

☐ Do I need a second opinion?

☐ Have I looked into gathering information from credible health/medical blogs, online groups and forums?

14

How to Get Discounted Medical Care and Discounted Medications

"I negotiated some costs with a highly recommended urologist, including the cost of pathology that would be involved. I got his estimates in writing. When the pathology bill came in thousands of dollars over the urologist's estimate, I simply sent a copy of the estimate to the pathologist and said that it would be unethical to charge me more unless he had done something unusual, which I knew he had not. That's the last I heard from the pathologist. I know what it costs to do pathology and the bill from the pathologist was outrageous."

JOHN T. JAMES, PHD, PATIENT SAFETY AMERICA, HOUSTON, TX

Discounted Medical Care

Many people don't think they can negotiate their medical bills. You can negotiate the purchase of a car or home and you can also negotiate with your doctor or hospital about your medical costs. If you decide to negotiate, you may not be able to use a credit card.

Many doctors who don't take health insurance offer a 20 percent discount if you pay their bill in the first thirty days. Most don't divulge that information. Ask your doctor's nurse or front office person if the doctor offers this discount.

"My advice for patients without insurance is to discuss payment options before medical treatment or a procedure is performed. Unfortunately, if the patient already has some form of health insurance, then the hospital or physician may be obligated by contract (between the health care provider and the patient) as determined by the insurance, to charge their regular fee."

Jack C. Rosenfeld, MD,
Family Medicine and Geriatrics,
Lansdale, PA

Some doctors said that if they don't take Medicare, they will offer a reduced fee to Medicare patients. It can't hurt to ask.

Ask for a Cash Pay Discount

You can always ask your doctor, medical center, surgery center or hospital for a "cash pay" discount. Try to negotiate with all of these professionals and institutions ahead of time. Explain your situation and simply ask if you can receive a discount if you pay cash.

Wouldn't you prefer to receive payment in cash rather than haggling with insurance companies to get paid? Doctors and medical institutions would too.

Learn How to Negotiate

"I had a patient, a single mother who was fired from her job and was unable to afford COBRA. Her child developed appendicitis and after the surgery she negotiated a cash price with all the providers."

Jack C. Rosenfeld, MD,
Family Medicine and Geriatrics, Lansdale, PA

If you have health insurance, it is less likely that you can negotiate a discount on your medical care but it's worth a try. Your insurance company is already involved and cutting fees. Insurance companies get discounts of 30 to 40 percent or more and you can fight for the same discount.

If you do not have health insurance, you are in a position to negotiate a cash pay discount. If you are paying cash, you are probably being billed at a higher rate than an insurance company.

When you negotiate, you need to do so with a calm and polite but firm manner. Arguing or belittling the person you are negotiating with will only backfire. Prepare for negotiations as you would for a business meeting.

If you negotiate a discount and a payment plan, you must be prepared to pay on time or the negotiation has been wasted.

Start by finding the decision maker for the doctor's practice or medical facility. You might approach the doctor or the manager of a large doctor's practice or the finance manager of a hospital. Write down that person's name and contact information. Take notes on the conversation.

The time to negotiate is before you have the procedure, treatment, surgery, etc., not after, if you can help it. Explain to the hospital or doctor why you cannot pay the total fee. Explain your circumstances in simple, concrete language, such as, "The doctor's fee exceeds my monthly income. I will not have enough money to pay my rent and other expenses for my children. Here is what I can afford." And then quote a number that is less than you can afford and expect some negotiation.

When shopping for reduced fees for medical care in advance of your procedure or surgery, approaching the negotiation process in a confident manner is very important. However, if you are negotiating after the fact, several patient advocates say that it is important to be honest about why you cannot afford to pay the fees.

> "We came to the U.S. from France to visit family. The evening of our arrival in Chicago, my partner had a seizure. She was rushed to the hospital and was diagnosed with a brain tumor. Immediately we had to decide where to go for medical care. Going back to France was not an option. We decided to set up residence in the U.S. for my partner's surgery, radiation and chemotherapy.
>
> I became my partner's full time advocate and caregiver. Since we did not have health insurance, for a time she was a cash patient.
>
> A friend's father had been a hospital administrator. He gave me a crash course on how hospital finance works. What I learned was:
>
> • The doctors know little or nothing about how patients pay or how much things cost. I learned quickly it was not the physicians I would be dealing with to negotiate medical fees.
>
> • Identify all of the medical professionals who expect to get paid for any medical encounter (surgeon, hospital facility, anesthesiologist, etc.). Depending on the facility, they may have their own invoicing procedures.

> • *For each of them, find out who is the decision maker with whom you should be talking to start the negotiation process.*
>
> *I ended up at the head of finance at a major hospital. What I had been told was to ask how much the surgery and hospital stay would cost and then to offer 40% less than the initial price.*
>
> *I said this to the head of finance at the hospital:*
> • *We are going to be a cash patient.*
> • *There is no credit card.*
> • *Financing is not an option.*
> • *I will pay you by check when the medical treatment begins.*
>
> *I found out that if they are paid upfront as opposed to by an insurance company, there are no delays and no collection issues.*
>
> *It was just like negotiating for a car. I offered 40% of their fee. They countered with a figure, then I countered with a figure.*
>
> *We finally agreed on a 25-30% discount of the initial quote.*
>
> *I know it doesn't sound like healthcare is negotiable, but I know it is. It's been ten years and my partner is healthy and cancer free."*

Sarah, Advocate for the Patient, St. Louis, MO

If you are not comfortable negotiating, you can contact one of the organizations listed at the end of this chapter. Some will charge a percentage of the amount they saved you and others will bill at an hourly rate.

Ask for a Payment Plan

You can always ask for a payment plan. I did. When I found out that one of the specialists I saw for a procedure sent tissue samples to a pathology lab that charged me $2,500, I called the lab. First I asked for a discount. This was refused because my insurance company had already gotten involved.

I then asked for a payment plan and told the person I spoke to at the pathology lab what I could afford on a monthly basis. She agreed. There was no interest rate and no additional fee.

If you talk to your doctor and explain that you are having trouble financially, she may be able to arrange payment plans for you. The same goes for hospitals, surgery centers and other medical services.

If you've lost your health insurance, talk to your doctor. There may be someone in her office who can offer resources to help you.

Get the Best Price for Surgery

A few doctors said to inform the hospital or surgery center that you are paying cash and that you would like a discount. Tell them how much you can afford.

If you have health insurance, make sure that the surgeon, anesthesiologist and surgery center or hospital accept your insurance. Also determine whether your insurance will cover the entire surgery or a good portion of it. Don't forget that money isn't the only issue. You want the best surgeon possible.

If you can afford it, you can find the best surgeon without a thought to whether insurance covers this doctor's fee. If you pay cash, you can negotiate a discount. Not all doctors will do that, but it's worth a try.

Personally, if money were no object, I would go with the best surgeon I could find and not shop around. However, that isn't a reality for many of us. You can also use your research to negotiate a price with your doctor, surgery center or hospital.

Tips to Find the Best Price

- You can compare prices on websites such as HealthCareBlueBook. com. These websites provide information about average costs for medical care.

- The Health Care Blue Book also offers links to state agencies that monitor the quality of health care.

Tips to Find Discounted Medications

If you cannot afford the medication your doctor prescribes for you, talk to her. Be honest with her about your financial situation so she can help you. For example, you can ask, "Is there a less expensive alternative?"

Please don't be embarrassed to let your doctor know that you cannot afford the medication she prescribed. Doctors are used to hearing this and they can come up with options for you.

- Some doctors suggested asking for a higher dose of medication so you can split the pill in half.

- Your doctor may give you free samples of medications. These free samples can be a wonderful gift if you have a time-limited illness or disease. Doctors get free samples from pharmaceutical companies and they pass them on to you.

   If you need this medication for longer than the samples last, know that you will have to figure out a way to get more medication. All samples are "brand" medication.

- Ask your physician for resources for free medications from pharmaceutical companies.

- If you are prescribed a new medicine, don't hesitate to ask your doctor what your out-of-pocket expense will be. If your doctor doesn't know, call your pharmacist. She will know the price of the medication and how much your health insurance will cover.

- If you want less expensive medications, look for generic drugs at major drug store chains, as they may be less expensive than smaller pharmacies.

- See if your state offers a discounted drug program.

- Check these private groups that offer prescription assistance:
   - Chronic Disease Fund
     http://www.cdfund.org/patient/apply.aspx
   - FamilyWize
     http://www.familywize.com/
   - Healthwell Foundation
     http://www.healthwellfoundation.org/
   - NeedyMeds
     http://www.needymeds.org/
   - Partnership for Prescription Assistance
     https://form.pparx.org/selectmedication.php
   - RxAssist
     http://www.rxassist.org/search/default.cfm
   - RxHope
     https://www.rxhope.com/patient/medsearchhome.aspx

Medical Care for Less

Community Health Centers and Federally Funded Health Centers

There are community health centers and federally qualified health centers across the country that provide health care to low-income people and those who do not have health insurance. There are more than 3,000 community health centers in the United States.

If you do not have health insurance, you will be charged a fee for service on a sliding scale based on your income. Community health centers provide ongoing care and health management for individuals and families. They are staffed by physicians, nurses, dentists and other medical professionals and volunteers.

They offer

- primary care visits,
- health education,
- disease control and screening,
- laboratory services,
- dental care,
- pharmacy services,
- and much more.

Many offer day, evening and weekend appointments and many employ multilingual staffs.

You can start by looking up community health centers online or go to http://www.nachc.org.

The Department of Health and Human Services provides assistance through federally funded health centers (http://bphc.hrsa.gov/). You pay what you can afford based on your income level. Their services include everything from preventative care to dental work.

Retail Medical Clinics

If you do not have a serious medical issue, you can visit a retail medical clinic (such as Minute Clinic inside CVS pharmacies). They can be less expensive than going to your primary care doctor. For additional information on retail medical clinics, please see Chapter 19.

Resources

Organizations That Help You Find Affordable Insurance and Free Health Care

- Patient Advocate Foundation
  http://www.patientadvocate.org/help4u.php

- Coverage For All
  http://www.coverageforall.org/

- Foundation For Health Coverage Education
  http://www.coverageforall.org/

Companies that Negotiate Your Medical Bills

- Medical Cost Advocates
  http://www.medicalcostadvocate.com/

- Health Advocate
  http://www.healthadvocate.com/

PATIENT CHECKLIST

☐ Do I understand how to negotiate a cash pay discount?

☐ Do I understand how to negotiate my medical bills?

☐ Do I want to ask for a payment plan?

☐ If I need less expensive medications, do I understand the options for finding them?

☐ Do I need to go to a community health center or government-funded health center?

15

Your Health Insurance

"The most common problem for patients is when they don't realize they have out-of-pocket expenses for their medical bills. It's surprising that people pay their premiums only to find out they have horrendous deductibles. People need to be more educated about what health plan they are purchasing."

LINDA E. KAY, MEDICAL BILLER, CULVER CITY, CA

Before you gloss over this chapter because it screams boredom, think about this: if you don't understand your health insurance plan, in all likelihood you will be stuck with medical bills you didn't plan on.

This chapter contains simple steps and basic instruction on how to get a handle on your health insurance plan and what to do if your medical treatment is denied. This is the most basic information you need to know but it does not cover everything.

"When you most need it, it becomes an issue. At that point, patients say, 'I wish I'd chosen another health insurance plan.'"

Zouhdi A. Hajjaj, MD,
Internal Medicine,
Yarmouthport, MA

Understanding Your Health Insurance Plan

It is difficult for most of us to understand our health insurance plans.

Health insurance plans can be confusing and they can change at any time. Even though it's a real challenge, you need to understand the basics.

"Patients must take some responsibility. If you buy a new TV, you'll take the time to read the instructions. This is your health care."

Linda E. Kay, Medical Biller,
Culver City, CA

This is very important. Too many patients find out after the fact that their tests, procedures or surgeries are not covered by their health insurance. Find out before. You must know your plan.

Know the answers to these questions before you see your doctor, other medical professional or are admitted to a hospital:

- What is my co-pay?

- What is my deductible?

- Are my doctor, other medical professional and hospital/surgery center covered by my health insurance plan?

- Am I seeing in-network providers? If not, how much will an out-of-network provider cost? Will my health insurance plan pay anything if I see a doctor who does not take insurance?

- Does my plan cover prescription medication?

- Does my health insurance cover nurse practitioners and physician's assistants?

- Does my plan cover acupuncture, physical therapy, and other therapies?

- If I have primary and secondary insurance, do I understand what each one covers?

- If I have an HMO, does it allow me to choose the doctors I want to see?

- Do I understand what Medicare covers? Does it include the doctors I wish to see? Which hospitals/surgery centers will it cover?

- Does my plan cover me if I travel outside of the United States?

If you receive health insurance through your employer, you can ask your human resources department for information.

If you call your health insurance company to get answers to these or other questions, be sure to write down the name of the person you speak to, the date, the time and the answers she gives you. It is very important to keep detailed notes.

Choosing a Primary Care Physician

Choose a primary care physician who is in network and is covered by your health insurance plan. If you can afford it, you can see a doctor out of network or a doctor who does not take your health insurance, but you will have to pay additional fees. Even if you see a doctor who does not take your insurance, you can submit your superbills (a superbill is the bill you receive for a visit with your doctor or other medical professional) and possibly get partial reimbursement.

> "Patients need to understand their insurance policies, guidelines and benefits. They need to know their insurance financial obligations, liabilities, deductibles and out-of-pocket expenses. This is a long-term process and relationship. Patients need to know how to contact their insurance company, know their rights and what they are entitled to. Many insurance claims are processed offshore. You may be dealing with people at insurance companies where English is their second language."
>
> J.C., Patient Advocate, Santa Monica, CA

How to Submit Your Health Insurance Claims

If your doctor or other medical professional does not do this for you, you must submit your own claim.

You should receive a superbill at the end of your visit with your doctor or other medical professional. Make a copy of your superbill and place it in your health insurance file.

> "Most of the billing complaints I receive involve out-of-network charges from insurance companies. Patients don't understand their benefits. They assume everything will be covered by their insurance company."
>
> Anonymous Medical Office Manager, Miami, FL

- Make a copy of your health insurance card.

- Download the claim form from your health insurance company's website or obtain a claim form in some other way.

Make copies of the blank claim form. Keep them in your health insurance file so that you will have them for future use.

- Fill out the claim form and attach it to your superbill. Attach a copy of your health insurance card.

- Send your claim to your health insurance company certified with a return receipt requested.

Review Your Explanation of Benefits (EOB)

You know those forms that come in the mail from your health insurance company that say "Explanation of Benefits" at the top of the page? You do need to read those. I know, no one reads them, right? Boring! I didn't read them either until I had a medical condition that forced me to see doctors and undergo medical procedures, treatments, tests and more. I started receiving a number of EOBs in the mail. I started reading them. I called my health insurance company when I didn't understand them and I was surprised to find out that most of the time the customer service representatives were really helpful.

Why It Is Important to Review Your EOBs

Your medical bills could contain errors. Check the EOB for your correct name, the doctor you saw, what you were billed for and your ID number. Just recently I discovered an error on one of my EOBs. When I called my health insurance company, I had my EOB in hand so I had access to all of the necessary information. The customer service representative admitted the error, said she noted it, and also said I should be receiving a check within the next week.

Before I had my medical condition, I threw my EOBs away. Now I understand just how important they are and I keep them in my health file. Sound like a chore? It is. But you could save yourself money like I did.

If your EOB shows bundled charges that you don't understand, call the customer service number on your health insurance card and ask questions.

Your EOBs may also include information about your prescription drug plan coverage. If there are changes to your plan, they may be shown in your EOB. If you are taking a medication that is no longer covered by your health insurance company, your EOB may reflect that or you will be informed by letter.

Your EOBs also serve as evidence of medical expenses for your taxes. It's good to keep them in a file in case you should need documentation.

Dealing with the Denial of a Health Insurance Claim

What to Do If Your Claim Is Denied

Many people are taken by surprise when their insurance company denies a claim.

If this happens to you, start by getting organized. Call your doctor's office. Ask to speak to the medical biller or to the person who takes care of billing. Request her assistance.

> "Insurance companies are going to try to deny a service. You have the right to appeal."
>
> Linda E. Kay, Medical Biller, Culver City, CA

You must be part of the process. Create a paper trail of everyone you speak to. Take copious notes on every conversation you have about the denial. Include names, dates and times.

Jackie Koob, RN, a senior reviewer for the grievance and appeals department of a major health insurance company, said that many insurance companies are now sending claim processing and customer service offshore. She suggested that in addition to getting the name of the person you speak with, ask for the "tracking number of your call in the system" and the employee ID number. Many states require that insurance companies have a tracking system to log member calls and concerns. That tracking number is the easiest way to refer someone back to your original call if you should need to do so.

Some Reasons for Claim Denials:

- Many insurance denials occur because of an administrative error. It may be that you can get this issue resolved by one phone call or a letter sent by certified mail, return receipt requested.

- Many denials are made simply because of missing data. Go over your patient information for accuracy, and ask your doctor to check diagnosis and procedure codes for accuracy.

- Your claim will be denied if your health insurance plan doesn't cover what your doctor ordered for you. You need to find out if it's a justified denial. If you don't have the booklet that came with your health insurance plan, call the customer service number and ask questions. Write down the name of the person you spoke to and the date, and take notes on what she said. If you have Medicare, you can also go to the Medicare website for help.

- If you have two insurance plans, make sure your doctor knows which insurance company to bill. Errors can be caused by the wrong insurance being billed.

How to Appeal a Denial

If you have a problem that is not a simple error but a true denial of your claim, you can file an appeal.

Each insurance plan has its own set of rules about time limits for submitting an appeal. Make sure you follow your plan's procedure, especially about how much time you have to submit an appeal.

Based on the requirements in your state and of your individual health plan, you may have to start with a phone call, followed by a letter. If a letter is necessary, send it certified with return receipt requested to make sure you have a record of it being sent and received.

> "It's up to the patient to stay on top of this—call the doctor and see if he's done what he needs to do and then call the insurance company and find out if they've received what they've requested. The doctor or patient (whoever is faxing records) should get a fax receipt to prove the insurance company received their records. I recommend that the doctor or patient get the name of a specific person at the insurance company to fax the necessary information to and put a cover sheet on their medical records and/or forms containing the name of that person."
>
> Fran Ginsberg, Medical Office Manager,
> Santa Monica, CA

Tips:

- Ask for your doctor's help in making your case. Ask your doctor to contact your health insurance company.
- Save all copies of your paperwork from your doctor.
- Try to deal with a supervisor at your insurance company and deal directly with this person each time you call.

- Make sure all your calls to the insurance company are documented. Write down the name of the person you spoke to, the date and time and the details of the conversation. You must create a paper trail. You get more attention that way and the insurance company knows you are serious.

- According to several professional medical billers, insurance companies seem to listen more when their contractual obligations are brought to their attention. This will be easier for you to do if you understand your plan.

Believe me, I am not giving you this information because it's interesting or fun. It's just very important and necessary. I have to deal with health insurance issues too. I no longer ignore my EOBs when they arrive in the mail, no longer throw all things health insurance in a drawer and never look at them. I learned the hard way because like a lot of people, I thought I'd never get sick and would never have to deal much with my health insurance plan.

Boy, was I wrong.

I had to go through all of my superbills and submit them. I had to call my doctors' offices and find out which had submitted my bills. I had to call and negotiate my medical bills, file claims and appeals—the works. I wish I had been on top of things before I got sick. If I could turn back the clock now, I would have handled my health insurance very differently. I would have chosen a different health insurance plan, I would have reviewed my EOBs and I would have taken the time to learn before I really needed my health insurance to kick in.

So, I tell you all of this because I don't want you to fall into the same trap.

What to Do If Your First Appeal is Denied

- Call the person who handles medical billing in your doctor's office and ask for help.

- Call your health insurance company's customer service number. Request a formal review by the insurance company. Ask the customer service representative to explain the necessary steps. Write them down. Ask for her name and write it down, along with the date and time you spoke.

- State your case for appeal in writing and send the letter certified mail with return receipt requested.

- If your health insurance company claims that the cost of your care is above their customary cost, request to see the doctor's notes. These notes may show that there are extenuating circumstances in your case that justify the additional cost. Ask your doctor if she has any additional information that could support your appeal. Make sure you have everything in writing. Make sure you have copies of everything.

What You Can Do as a Last Resort

> "We spend so much time in medical school and in residency, learning so much, and now insurance companies are running our practices. We feel so knowledgeable about how to deliver good medical care and now we are so restricted. We are caught in the middle. There is nothing in medical school or residency that prepares us to navigate insurance issues. Doctors generally are not good business people. We know the right things to do medically and then the insurance company denies it."
>
> Sheryl A. Ross, MD,
> Obstetrics and Gynecology, Santa Monica, CA

If you have exhausted your insurance company's appeal process or your insurance plan does not respond, contact the office of your state's department of insurance. Every state has a different way of helping patients with health insurance appeals.

You can also request an independent external review. Your state's department of insurance will be able to tell you if your state offers this option.

How Health Insurance Affects Your Medical Care

> "Insurance companies deny things, need authorizations for everything which delays surgeries and treatments. This could compromise patient care and lead to friction between the doctor, the staff and the patient. Patients are puzzled and upset when they make the decision to have surgery and the surgery is delayed because of the insurance company."
>
> Rene Osman, MD, Urology, Northridge, CA

According to many doctors, health insurance prevents them from practicing the kind of medicine they were trained to do. It is very frustrating for so many of them to have tests, procedures, surgeries and medications denied because the patient's health insurance company says so. According to insurance companies they are trying to prevent unnecessary medical care and costs.

Your Annual Exam

You don't want to arrive at your doctor's office and find out you scheduled your annual physical too soon. You must schedule your appointment when it will be covered by your health insurance plan. Call your insurance company and find out before you make the appointment with the doctor.

Tests, Procedures and Surgeries

If your doctor recommends a test, procedure or surgery, her office staff may make all the necessary phone calls to find out what your health insurance covers. It is up to you to monitor your doctor's staff and their progress with getting authorization from your insurance carrier.

> "I have issues with the insurance companies. I had a patient who I had diagnosed with lymphoma. I ordered a CT scan which the insurance company denied. This frustrated me. I wrote a letter and then argued with the insurance company over the phone to appeal this denial. The fact that I had to appeal a CT scan is a waste of my time. I can't manage my patients the way I want."
>
> Michael C. Dobrow, DO,
> Family Medicine, Hoboken, NJ

Insurance companies may try to deny any number of tests, procedures and surgeries. They are trying to prevent unnecessary medical care and skyrocketing costs. Their goal is to save money and prevent unnecessary tests, procedures, surgeries and treatments.

Surgery Centers

Some surgery centers aren't covered by your insurance. Just because a doctor suggests a surgery center for your procedure doesn't mean your insurance will pay for it. If your

> "Administrative work is 20% of my workload now. I spend time pleading with insurance companies for an MRI for a patient. The system is set up to reject expensive diagnostic imaging. I have to tell patients to call the Member Services number on their health insurance card to see if the treatment plan I suggest is acceptable."
>
> Anonymous MD, New York, NY

"We spend so much time on the phone dealing with prior authorizations. The office staff is being utilized to full capacity because we are doing so much more than we were years ago, such as authorizations for drugs. Patients may have been on medications for years and now insurance companies are denying them because of formularies. Insurance companies can pick on little things to delay authorizations."

Patti Morris, Office Manager, Medical Assistant, Los Angeles, CA

health insurance company denies coverage for a surgery center, talk to your doctor about it. Ask questions.

Your Medications
Your insurance company will have its own formulary of medications. This means they will allow or cover certain medications and not others. Don't be surprised if your doctor prescribes a medication for you and your insurance company will not pay for it. Your doctor's office may appeal the decision if your doctor thinks the medication is medically necessary, or she may suggest another medication that will work for you.

What to Do If Your Doctor Stops Taking Your Health Insurance
Doctors do stop taking health insurance plans. Not necessarily because they want to but because health insurance reimbursements have become so low that doctors can't make enough money to justify contracting with certain plans.

If your doctor stops taking your health insurance, she should notify you.

What to Do If You Lose Your Job
If you have lost your job or have reduced work hours, you may be eligible for COBRA, a program that enables you to keep your employer's health insurance. The monthly fee can be pricey. For more information, visit http://www.dol.gov/ebsa/cobra.html.

Using a Health Insurance Advocate
There are independent professionals and professional organizations to help you with all of this. They work for you, not for health insurance companies. Many will provide assistance with issues involving medical debt, insurance access, job retention, medical billing, medical insurance claims, fee

"People should have a good insurance broker and go over their health plan frequently."   Kenneth Elconin, MD, Orthopedic Surgery, Beverly Hills, CA

negotiation, and much more. You can Google "health insurance advocates" and come up with a list. I am not recommending these organizations, simply providing you with information so you can do your own research.

Resources to Help You

- Patient Advocate Foundation (PAF)
- Healthcare Advocates, Inc.
- The Patient's Advocate
- The AHRQ (Agency for Healthcare Research and Quality) has information about how to choose a health plan. http://www.ahrq. gov/consumer/qualcare.html#plans

PATIENT CHECKLIST

☐ Do I understand my health insurance plan?

☐ Do I understand my co-pay and deductible?

☐ Is my doctor or hospital covered by my health insurance plan?

☐ Does my health insurance plan cover prescription medication?

☐ Does my health insurance plan cover alternative medicine or physical therapy?

☐ If I have lost my job, am I eligible for COBRA?

☐ If I have primary and secondary insurance, do I understand what each one covers?

☐ If I have an HMO, does it allow me to choose the doctors I want to see?

☐ Am I familiar with my EOBs?

☐ Do I need to submit a health insurance claim or does my doctor's office do that for me?

☐ If my health insurance claim has been denied, do I understand what my next steps are?

☐ Do I need to hire a health insurance advocate to help me?

16

Serious Illnesses and Chronic Medical Conditions

"If a patient has a serious illness, they enter a whole new world. This includes language, terminology, and shocking material to absorb."

DAVID A. RAPKIN, PHD, CLINICAL AND HEALTH PSYCHOLOGIST,
MIND-BODY MEDICINE GROUP, DIVISION OF HEAD AND NECK SURGERY,
UCLA DAVID GEFFEN SCHOOL OF MEDICINE, LOS ANGELES, CA

I was hesitant to write a chapter on serious illnesses or chronic medical conditions as there is so much information you need to know. There are entire books written on these subjects and I encourage you to seek them out.

If you have a serious illness or chronic medical condition, it can take a toll on your emotional health as well as your physical health. It can be a challenging time and it may be difficult for you to ask for help. If you haven't asked for help already, know that your loved ones want to assist you. Think about it: If your spouse, loved one or close friend had a serious illness or medical condition, would you not want to help her? Try to allow others to assist and care for you.

Get an Advocate

If you have a serious medical illness or medical condition, you must enlist the help of a family member, good friend or professional patient advocate. You may not think that you will need someone like this, but most patients do. Even patients without serious illnesses need advocates. Not because you're inept or cannot do the job yourself, but because the emotional and physical stress that accompany a medical condition affect how you will manage your treatments, side effects, conversations with doctors, medications, health insurance and much more.

> "A patient should choose an advocate. This person needs to be good at managing frustration."
>
> David A. Rapkin, PhD, Clinical and Health Psychologist, Mind-Body Medicine Group, Division of Head and Neck Surgery, UCLA David Geffen School of Medicine, Los Angeles, CA

Dealing with a serious medical illness causes stress. Stress interferes with cognitive function. You can ask a loved one to act as your advocate or enlist the help from several loved ones to act as a team of advocates for you.

You can also hire a professional patient advocate to help you navigate the medical system. Chapter 22 provides information on professional patient advocates.

Qualities of a Good Advocate

A good advocate should be

- diplomatic

- a good communicator

- well organized

- attentive to details

- willing to do research

- appreciative but assertive with medical professionals

> "We know from research that once the word cancer is spoken, that people retain about 20% of information that is told to them."
>
> Anne Coscarelli, PhD, Director, Simms/Mann-UCLA Center for Integrative Oncology, Los Angles, CA

I've been an advocate for loved ones, and believe me, there are many gifts in giving. Even though it was not easy being an advocate for my mother and godmother, who were seriously ill and in hospitals for extended stays and died in those hospitals, I would not have traded what I did for anything. It gave me a chance to give back for all they had given me. Being involved in their care also gave me a sense of control. Standing by when a loved one has a serious illness or medical condition isn't easy, but most people want to help in some way. Try to remember that if accepting help is difficult for you.

I have also been in a position when my pain was at its peak and I had seen too many doctors who could not find an accurate diagnosis and treatment plan. It was at a time of complete desperation and I could no longer handle everything myself when I asked a good friend who is medically savvy to be my advocate. In addition to my husband and a couple of close friends who were very supportive of me, I chose F. because she was very smart, understood medical language, had experience managing medical practices and was very caring and supportive. It was not easy for me to ask her. I have always considered myself to be strong, both physically and emotionally (not to mention controlling), so asking someone to help me was out of character. F. agreed. I offered to pay her. She refused. She said her payment was to see me get well and become pain free. She wanted to see me get my life back. I am very grateful to her to this day and would return the favor and act as her advocate in a heartbeat.

Not everyone has one person they feel comfortable asking to be their advocate. You can create an "advocate team"—two or more loved ones who pitch in as your support team throughout your illness or medical condition.

I didn't just have F. My husband and a few close friends were also a part of my support system. I am grateful to each one of them for being there for me while I was sick.

Give yourself permission to ask for help. You'll be glad you did. You can ask your advocate to

- take you to appointments with your doctors;
- take you to treatments, surgeries or procedures;
- sit with you while you meet with medical professionals and act as a second set of eyes and ears. You might not remember everything your doctor tells you if you are not feeling well;
- take notes on conversations with your doctors;

> "It's important for patients to evaluate motivation and availability of family and friends. Someone might really want to help but he/she lives 3000 miles away. Think through what tasks need to be done and who is best to do them. Assess the suitability of a person's skills to what you are asking them to do."
>
> David A. Rapkin, PhD, UCLA David Geffen School of Medicine, Los Angeles, CA

- go through your health file, health summaries, lists of medications, medical records and more, to make sure you have the essential information to take with you to your appointments with doctors and other medical professionals;

- help you research your diagnosis, doctors, treatment plans, medical facilities, medications and more;

- talk with you about your illness or medical condition to help you distill information you have heard;

- sort through your medications to make sure each one is what you are supposed to be taking;

- and much more.

What to Do When You're Given a Serious Diagnosis

If you've been given a serious diagnosis, you'll no doubt need time and support to process the information. Here are a number of steps to help you. Start doing what you can now.

As I said earlier, please gather other information on your illness as the information in this chapter simply isn't enough.

"Most people when faced with serious medical conditions find that they get in touch with a tremendous resiliency that is innate in human beings. Part of our survival skills is the ability to be flexible in the face of challenging and life-threatening situations. Illness activates this survival response, driving us to look at the world in new ways, to learn new ways of living which are more purposeful and meaningful, as well as connect with others and life in new ways which actually not only improve our lives, but can impact the illness itself. We become more mindful of what is precious. A major illness once thought terrible, can have a hidden treasure of gold in making our lives better."

Roger E. Dafter, PhD, Associate Director,
Mind-Body Medicine Group,
Division of Head and Neck Surgery,
UCLA David Geffen School of Medicine,
Los Angeles, CA

Create Your Support System

If you have a serious illness, you will need to create a support system. Not just for you, but if you have a spouse and children, they will need support as well. For example: if you cannot drive the kids to their after-school activities, will your spouse do the extra driving or can you count on a family member or good friend?

According to a few health psychologists, family and friends want to do a lot.

Create a Secondary Support System

You'll need a secondary support system for your immediate family. For example: You are a mother with two kids and you have cancer. You currently take care of your kids and when you are undergoing chemotherapy treatments, let's say your spouse takes over. Who supports your spouse while you are recuperating? Ask your advocate to help you figure this out.

Find a Health Psychologist

If you are able to see a therapist, preferably a health psychologist, you'll be happy you did. If you have a serious diagnosis, there are many sources of information and support that an experienced therapist can help you with. A health psychologist can help you sort through your concerns and questions about your illness or condition. Also, it can be very helpful to have someone listen to you who is not personally involved in your illness or condition.

> "If you get a diagnosis that is upsetting, make sure you schedule a follow-up appointment. You may not be able to think of all the questions at the time of diagnosis and more time may be needed to process what you've been told. For that follow-up appointment, bring in a list of questions. If you are unable to see the physician in person, schedule a follow-up phone call."
>
> Theodora Pinnock, MD, Developmental and Behavioral Pediatrics, Nashville, TN

Some health psychologists also function as professional advocates.

Take Care of Your Emotional Health

If you have a serious illness or chronic medical condition, several doctors suggested the importance of getting therapeutic support to help you deal with it. Processing what you are going through with a trained professional can be an important part of healing. Seeing a therapist does not mean you are weak. In my opinion, it shows strength to reach out for help from a professional.

> "I've had patients who have gone through radical treatments who have used those experiences to make enormous psychological breakthroughs."
>
> David A. Rapkin, PhD, UCLA David Geffen School of Medicine, Los Angeles, CA

It's not uncommon for depression, hopelessness, anxiety, anger, and other feelings to accompany a serious illness or medical condition. This can be a challenging time in your life. Reach out to trusted loved ones and ask for their support.

Join a Support Group

Consider finding a support group of people who share your medical condition or illness. You can exchange information and resources with other members. It will help you to connect with people who are going through what you are. You can find out about good doctors and treatments from members of the support group. You can also learn about clinical trials that other members are participating in and explore side effects, treatment and outcome.

Start by doing what you can now.

Develop Support Networks

As part of your journey, you may want to gather support from your loved ones and also share your progress with family and friends without calling or emailing each one individually. There are many opportunities for people who are experiencing a significant health challenge and want to connect to their loved ones.

For example, Caring Bridge (www.caringbridge.org) and CarePages (www.carepages.com) offer private space where you can post your story, along with updates on your health, photos and more, for your family and friends. They can leave messages for you. These sites have been developed to be easy to set up and are user friendly. You control access to your pages, so they can be as private or public as you wish.

Meal Train (www.mealtrain.com) makes it easy for you or your advocate to organize the delivery of meals when you need them. Your friends and family sign up to prepare meals, the menu is available for all to see, and you can list dietary restrictions and preferences.

Phone trees are another way to let your loved ones know when you have tests and results and want to provide updates on your progress and other information. After you create a list of people you want to include on the tree, you can assign a point person to whom you give the information you want passed on. She calls x number of people on the list and updates them as you have requested. They, in turn, contact x more people, and so on.

Create Your Health File

Put together your health file now. Please see Chapter 3 for information on what a health file is, what it contains and how to go about putting it together.

> "The only reliable way chronically ill patients can maintain power and control over their lives is to get copies of their medical records from all doctors and hospitals. Buy a scanner. Keep your files updated. Come prepared to meet the doctor."
>
> Michael A. Weiss, Author, Patient Advocate, West Orange, NJ

Your health file will include copies of your pertinent medical records, test results, copies and reports of MRIs and other scans, a list of your current medications and their dosages, and a list of over-the-counter medications, including herbs and supplements. It will contain names and contact information for doctors you see for your current illness or condition. Describe any alternative medicine treatments you are undergoing and name the practitioners you see.

Not only will this allow your doctors to see your medical history and current medical status, but it will also give you a sense of control.

By taking charge of your medical records and information, you are empowering yourself and becoming a take-charge patient. Take-charge patients feel more confident, less helpless and less vulnerable to the medical system they are dependent upon.

Create a Medical Journal

Going through a serious illness or chronic medical condition requires a steep learning curve on your part, as you will be learning a new language and how to navigate a new world. Taking notes on new doctors, terminology, possible treatments, new research, possible medications and more can help keep you organized and focused.

Your medical journal is also for keeping track of your symptoms and side effects, creating questions for your doctors, noting answers to your questions, and for anything you think of regarding your condition that you might want to refer to later.

Empower Yourself as a Take-Charge Patient

> "Control what you can regarding your medical care or else your 'uncontrollable' chronic illness will take away your confidence and thus your optimum ability to cope and manage the illness properly."
>
> Michael A. Weiss, Author,
> Patient Advocate, West Orange, NJ

If you are diagnosed with a serious illness or chronic medical condition, part of your battle is to maintain hope, confidence and a sense of control. *Control* is the key word because the more you can control as a patient, the more empowered you feel.

Tips for Becoming Empowered

- Create your health file with copies of all of your current medical records.

- Write your current health summary (see Chapter 3).

- Create your medical journal.

- Research doctors you need to see. If you are inexperienced with the internet, enlist a computer-savvy person to help you.

- Research recommended treatment plans.

- Create a support system of loved ones to help and support you.

- Create a buddy system. Pick a couple of good friends, family members or your spouse to help you distill medical information and generate ideas on how to seek good treatment.

- Become affiliated with a disease association such as the American Cancer Society. It can offer you information, resources and support. Such associations are devoted to empowering patients by providing the best information possible. You can obtain information from these organizations about online or in-person support groups.

- Don't put off what you can do now in regard to medical treatment.

- Join support groups for your medical condition.

- Research medications that are prescribed for you. Find out about their side effects, what they are for, what they will do and more. Discuss any questions you have with your doctor.

- Even if you are seeing a specialist, such as an oncologist, keep your PCP in the loop. Tell her about what medical treatments you are undergoing, which new medications you are taking and how you are doing. Your PCP should be aware of your treatment summary and your care plan.

- Keep a calendar for yourself. Keep track of dates for your next test, treatment or screening. If a doctor tells you that a certain test should happen within a certain amount of time, write it down and stay on top of it. Ask your doctor for a time line so you can stay organized.

- Prepare now. Preparing ahead of time is always easier than leaving it for later. If you are diagnosed with a serious illness or chronic medical condition, get organized now. Who will help you? Who will help your family? Which doctors might you see? Will you hire a professional advocate? Do you want to consult with your religious institution and see what they offer that may help? (For more information, see Chapter 21).

- Make connections now with people who will help serve your needs later on. Create a list of things you need to do in the next two weeks. Do you need therapeutic support? Do you need a health psychologist who specializes in supporting and advocating

"Disease progression is the biggest issue. When and if the patients come back and decide to become proactive, they may have fewer options which can be less successful."

Rene Osman, MD, Urology, Northridge, CA

"Educate yourself. Understand which medications you are on, what they do, how they work, side effects and down sides. Find out what side effects, especially from chemo, can be permanent. You have to have the confidence to challenge a doctor if you don't think what he's saying is correct. You have to listen to yourself."

Laura, Patient, Baltimore, MD

"We see very gravely ill patients, transplant patients and patients with serious diseases. The most successful patients are those who keep their appointments, take their medications, and follow up with the doctor. If there is a problem with their insurance that interferes with their medical care, they call me."

Patti Morris, Office Manager, Medical Assistant, Los Angeles, CA

"Become informed.
I say that cautiously
because the way people
can get informed can
be overwhelming.
Understand something
about your disease but
be careful to stay away
from statistics that can
be scary. They may not
apply to you."

Anne Coscarelli, PhD,
Director, Simms/Mann–
UCLA Center for Integrative
Oncology, Los Angles, CA

"Even if you have
complete confidence
in your doctor, get a
second opinion. It will
educate you. You'll get
to ask more questions.
This allows you to
determine if there
are other treatment
options. Often people
are frightened and want
to move fast. Getting
a second opinion can
radically change your
opinion of treatment or
radically confirm your
opinion."

Anne Coscarelli, PhD,
Director, Simms/Mann–
UCLA Center for Integrative
Oncology, Los Angles, CA

for people with your medical condition? If so, make the call now or at least write down a name with a note to research this later.

- Become very familiar with your health insurance plan. Some people have long-term care policies—find out if you have benefits to hire a home health aide. You may not need that, but it's so much easier to find out now when you are up to it.

- Research your illness. Use credible websites and check the information with your doctors.

- Jacki Koob, RN, suggested asking your insurance plan to assign a case manager to you. She explained that this person can help coordinate services and navigate around obstacles for care.

- Get a second opinion, and even a third. This is not just to confirm your diagnosis and possible treatment, but to instill confidence in you.

- Prioritize. Your time and energy are important now.

- Delegate responsibilities. The demands of treatment can be great, so take care of yourself and enlist your advocate and loved ones to help you at home.

- Get educated about side effects. Learn which are important and which are simply bothersome. Record side effects you experience in your medical journal. Keep track. Talk to your doctor about them. Bring in your medical journal when you meet with her.

Find the Right Specialist for You

When dealing with a chronic medical condition or serious illness, finding the best doctor for you is very important. Having the right specialist is important not only for your diagnosis and treatment, but also for your hope, faith and journey through the process. It is crucial for your confidence in your treatment. Find a specialist whom you feel very comfortable with. Several doctors suggested that in the case of a serious illness such as cancer, you must be able to talk to your doctor and tell her when you don't feel comfortable. One doctor suggested looking for "the warm fuzzy feeling" when considering an oncologist.

> "Patients with chronic or serious illnesses will have—as either side effects of treatments or as a direct result of the medical condition—issues such as pain, depression and anxiety, fatigue, loss of mental clarity, and other symptoms that can limit their functionality and affect their capacity to comply with their treatment regimes."
>
> David A. Rapkin, PhD, UCLA David Geffen School of Medicine, Los Angeles, CA

Chapter 4 contains all the strategies you need to find the best doctor for you. But in addition, you'll be looking for a physician who helps to instill confidence, hope and a sense of control over what is happening to your body. You will be participating in your medical care as an active team member regarding treatment decisions, medications, and sharing research with your doctor. It is essential for you to feel comfortable asking as many questions as you need to, reporting side effects, discussing possible alternative treatments and much more.

> "If a patient believes a treatment will work, there is a greater chance that it will."
>
> David A. Rapkin, PhD, UCLA David Geffen School of Medicine, Los Angeles, CA

Find a doctor who is comfortable with a take-charge patient.

If you haven't read Chapter 2 on what it means to be a take-charge patient, please do so.

Sample Questions to Ask Your Specialist

If you have a serious illness or chronic medical condition, the questions to ask your doctor are different than if you were seeing a doctor for a less serious medical issue.

> "Never go to a specialist's appointment alone. Virtually all patients have difficulty remembering what physicians say. Your buddy/advocate will take notes and keep track of your questions to ensure that the most important questions are posed to the physician early in the meeting."
>
> H. Kenneth Schueler, Professional Patient Advocate, New York, NY

You need to formulate questions before you see your specialist. Write down the answers in your medical journal. You'll want to refer to them later and possibly discuss them with other doctors and loved ones.

Here is a list of suggested questions to ask your specialist. This list is not all-inclusive. Please refer to books on your illness or chronic medical condition to learn about additional questions to ask.

- What is the stage of my disease?
- Are the causes of my medical condition known?
- What are the most successful treatments for my disease?
- Which doctors have successfully treated this type of disease?
- Who will be in charge of my treatment?
- What are the side effects of the treatment?
- What is the success rate of the treatment?
- Is there a consensus about what medical treatment is most effective for my condition? According to a health psychologist, having consensus doesn't mean that a treatment is necessarily the *right* treatment but that it is statistically more likely to work than others.
- Are there alternative treatments?
- If your doctor has given you a treatment plan, you can ask the following question, "Please help me understand why this is the best treatment for me."
- You can also ask your doctor, "If this were your diagnosis, what would you do next?"

How to Decide on a Treatment Plan

When faced with a treatment plan, you might feel an urgency to jump right in. This is perfectly understandable, but unless there is a medical necessity for starting the plan immediately, take a moment to reflect on it. You'll want to get a second opinion from another specialist, do your own research, talk about the options with your doctors and loved ones, and find out as much information as you can before you make a commitment.

Research the Proposed Treatment Plan

Research the proposed treatment plan on credible websites and discuss it with your doctor, other medical professionals, your loved ones and other patients who have gone through the same treatment. The more you know about a treatment, the more confident you will be as a patient. Knowledge is the best antidote to helplessness.

If you are not comfortable with researching, ask a loved one or friend to help you.

Please remember that anyone can create a website. Not all information on the internet is credible, and some of it can be downright scary. It may be tempting to simply Google your disease. Try to refrain from doing this.

> "If you have a serious illness, you'd better become your own specialist in your disease. Get informed."
>
> Linda Nadwodny, DO, FAAFP, Family Medicine, Lansdale, PA

Ask your specialist to refer you to websites she believes have information that would benefit you. Ask her for handouts and names of books. You can also see the Resources section at the end of this book.

Weigh the Benefits and Risks of a Treatment Plan

When presented with a treatment plan, you must decide whether you can follow what the doctor is suggesting. You must weigh the risks and benefits and how it will affect your quality of life now and in the long run. Ask if any of the treatments have lasting side effects.

You'll want to ask:

- What does the treatment consist of?
- What will I be going through?
- How long will it take and how often will I receive treatment?
- What are the side effects? Are any long lasting or permanent?

> "Ask yourself the question, 'At the end of this set of medical interventions, what is my quality of life going to be?'"
>
> Jessica G. Schairer, PhD, Clinical and Health Psychologist, Los Angeles, CA

- Will I need extra care at home?
- Will I be able to work?
- What are the costs of this treatment?
- Will my health insurance cover the cost?
- And more...

Get a Second Opinion

Even if you have complete confidence in the doctor who is proposing a treatment plan, get a second opinion from a doctor with the same specialty. Seek out a board-certified physician who is affiliated with a medical school and who specializes in the disease or medical condition you have.

> "Laura, my best friend of thirty-eight years, had stage-four terminal breast cancer. She was put on the chemotherapy drug Taxol. Tragically, she was not informed of the side effects of this drug, which included permanent neuropathy (painful tingling, burning and numbness in the feet). Her oncologist, who was on staff at a renowned teaching hospital, was out of the office for seven weeks due to back surgery. In her doctor's absence, a nurse practitioner (NP) was following her and many other patients who were getting chemo. Laura reported her side effects to the NP after her second treatment and continued to tell her that she was experiencing tingling, burning and numbness in her feet. The nurse ignored her symptoms and didn't report it to the physician overseeing the chemo patients. The neuropathy continued for the next six weeks, in which time she had three or four more doses of Taxol.
>
> Upon her oncologist's return, he realized Laura had neuropathy and immediately stopped the Taxol. The chemo-induced neuropathy was irreversible and there was no treatment for it. Laura tearfully told me, 'I had stage-four cancer and did not have the energy to challenge that nurse. I was in pain. I also had no idea the neuropathy would be permanent.'
>
> Laura died one year later. During the last year of her life, she had agonizing, debilitating pain from the neuropathy. As a result of the nerve damage and muscle weakness from the neuropathy, Laura

*was off balance and lost the ability to walk properly. She couldn't
feel her feet touch the ground and could only walk using a walker.
She became more depressed and couldn't sleep because of the
severe pain and constant tingling, burning, and numbness in her
feet."*

Carol, Friend of the Patient, Baltimore, MD

Use Support Groups to Gather Information

*"Because I have three cancers and Alpha-1 (Antitrypsin
Deficiency, an inherited emphysema that causes lung disease) I
am very active in support groups. I go to national conferences
on Alpha-1. I formed a support group for Alpha-1. I go to all the
educational meetings so I can to stay on top of the research."*

John O. Will, Patient, Horsham, PA

Whether online or in person, find support groups with members who
have the same disease or medical condition you have. If you aren't a group
type of person, at least consider communicating with other members to
gather information.

Talking with other patients who are dealing with your medical condition
is very important for many reasons.

You can learn about treatments that are available and which are working
for people. Members might share their opinions about the best specialists and
how to find them. You might also hear about what eases certain side effects
you are dealing with. In addition to providing essential information and
possibly a different perspective, support groups can be a source of comfort.

Ask About Alternatives to Treatment

Even if you are fairly certain you want to commit to a proposed medical
treatment, it is wise to ask about alternatives. You may not have considered
other options. Learning about other options for treatment will benefit you in
two ways: you might feel even more committed to your proposed treatment
or you might find alternatives that are better for you.

Always ask your PCP and specialist for their opinions on any other
options you consider.

Consider a Clinical Trial

"Clinical trials are generally considered to be biomedical or health-related research studies in human beings that follow a pre-defined protocol. ClinicalTrials.gov includes both interventional and observational types of studies. Interventional studies are those in which the research subjects are assigned by the investigator to a treatment or other intervention, and their outcomes are measured. Observational studies are those in which individuals are observed and their outcomes are measured by the investigators."

clinicaltrials.gov

Participants in clinical trials gain access to new research treatments before they are widely available and obtain expert medical care at leading health care facilities during the trial.

Depending on the kind of clinical trial being conducted, the research team includes doctors and nurses as well as social workers and other health care professionals. They work closely with the participants throughout the process. Participants follow specific instructions, and are monitored carefully during and after the trial.

Discuss Clinical Trials with Your Doctor

- At an office visit, ask your doctor if a clinical trial might be right for you. Your doctor knows you and your medical history. She can help you make an informed decision.

- Ask your doctor to help you get information about clinical trials and formulate important questions to ask prior to joining a clinical trial.

- Ask your doctor how to connect with other patients who are participating in clinical trials, such as through online forums or groups.

Steps to Finding a Clinical Trial

- Ask your PCP, specialist or nurse (or all three) if there is a clinical trial that might be right for you. Health care professionals have access to medical journals and online databases that provide information on clinical trials.

- Ask family members or friends to help you conduct a comprehensive search of clinical trials you might qualify for.

- Check a reputable disease website for a list of current clinical trials being conducted.

- Call local clinical research centers that specialize in your medical condition to obtain information about clinical trials. Research centers usually have websites and may be linked to academic health centers.

For more information, such as important questions to ask about clinical trials, please go to www.clinicaltrials.gov

If you join a clinical trial, you should continue to receive care from your primary care physician or specialist.

Resources for Clinical Trials

- http://www.cancer.gov/clinicaltrials/
- http://www.clinicaltrials.gov/
- http://www.searchclinicaltrials.org/

A Few Resources for Your Serious Illness or Chronic Medical Condition

Find a patient advocacy organization, disease organization or medical society dedicated to your medical condition or disease. Find groups of people, either online or in person, who share your disease or medical condition. Many doctors said that these are very helpful for chronic diseases such as diabetes.

- American Cancer Society
  http://www.cancer.org/

- Cancer Support Community
  http://www.cancersupportcommunity.org/

- The Lance Armstrong Foundation
  http://www.livestrong.org/

- Patient Access Network
  http://www.panfoundation.org/

- Patient Advocate Foundation
  http://www.patientadvocate.org/

- PBS.org—Who Cares: Chronic Illness in America
  http://www.pbs.org/inthebalance/archives/whocares/resources.html

- Stanford School of Medicine
  Chronic Disease Self-Management Program
  http://patienteducation.stanford.edu/programs/cdsmp.html

See the Resources section at the back of this book for more information.

PATIENT CHECKLIST

- ☐ Do I have an advocate?

- ☐ What will I ask my advocate to do for me?

- ☐ Have I created my primary and secondary support system?

- ☐ Do I need the support of a therapist?

- ☐ Did I look into joining a support group?

- ☐ Did I develop a support network?

- ☐ Is my health file up to date?

- ☐ Have I started my medical journal?

- ☐ Have I researched a specialist?

- ☐ Have I created a list of questions for the specialist?

- ☐ Have I researched my diagnosis?

- ☐ Have I researched my treatment plan and asked my doctors about benefits and risks?

- ☐ Does my health insurance cover my medical treatment?

- ☐ Did I talk to my primary care physician about my diagnosis and treatment plan?

- ☐ Did I get a second opinion?

17

Tests, Procedures and Surgeries

"I went into surgery because I want to fix people.
Most medical conditions are chronic.
I hate chronic disease. With surgery, you can fix it."

CHARLES A. HUNTER, MD, FACS, GENERAL SURGERY, LOS ANGELES, CA

No patient wants to have a test, procedure or surgery. But sometimes they are necessary. It's important that before you have them that you gather information so you can make an informed decision.

Partner with your doctor about decisions concerning tests, procedures and surgeries. Ask questions about the benefits and the risks of each. People who work with their doctors to make decisions about their medical care are more confident in the care they receive.

Every test, procedure or surgery will have benefits and risks. Find out from your doctor what they are and discuss them. Explore other sources as well and compare the information you uncover with what you have heard from your doctor. Discuss your findings with a loved one.

Educate yourself about your medical problem. Learn all you can from credible sources. You can ask your doctor for information on your medical condition. There are credible websites listed in the Resources section of this book. Your local library is also a good source of information. The librarian can help you find it.

Tests and Procedures

Screening tests are important because they can help protect against certain diseases. Some screening tests find diseases early when they are most treatable, while others can actually play a role in stopping diseases before they start. Please see Chapter 20 for more information on which screening tests you should have at what age.

If your doctor suggests that you have a test, find out ahead of time if your health insurance covers the test, the medical facility in which it will be conducted, and any medical professionals that might be involved.

Procedures can also be called medical tests but procedures can be medical interventions with the intent to treat a medical condition, injury or disease.

Risks of Tests

Some tests entail risks. The type and amount of risk varies from person to person and from test to test. What might be a risk for you might not be one for me. Risks depend on the test but also on your condition, your health history and a number of other factors. As a take-charge patient, work with your doctor to determine which tests are appropriate for you.

Test Results Can Be Inaccurate

"You can talk to your doctor if the test result doesn't fit the picture. Test results can be inaccurate. Your history and physical are the biggest part of the diagnosis."

Susan Tritt, MD, FACOG, Obstetrics and Gynecology, Santa Monica, CA

Test results can be inaccurate and show false positive or false negative results. This means that the test results could show something you do not have or they could miss something you do actually have. Ask questions. Speak up. You can request the test to be repeated or read by another medical professional.

"'Unfortunately, it's cancer.' Those words stunned me when I called my doctor for the biopsy results of a lump I had discovered in my left breast. Three months earlier, I'd had a mammogram and ultrasound, which were both clear. When I discovered this lump, I decided to have it checked just to be safe. I'm so glad I did. The tumor along with the two sentinel lymph nodes were removed

and the pathology results were positive with no further surgery required. I feel so lucky. If I hadn't been doing monthly self breast exams, a year would have gone by before this was discovered and the outcome may have been dramatically different."

Debbie Berman, Patient, Los Angeles, CA

Ask Questions

If your doctor, nurse practitioner or physician's assistant recommends a test or procedure, ask questions.

For example:

> "If your doctor cannot explain the procedure or surgery in a way you can understand, don't just accept it. Wait on moving forward until you do understand."
>
> Theodora Pinnock, MD,
> Developmental and
> Behavioral Pediatrics,
> Nashville, TN

- What is the test or procedure for?

- What could it show?

- Are there any downsides?

- Are there any side effects?

- Is this test covered by my health insurance?

- Is any preparation involved?

- Will I be able to drive home after this test?

- Do I need to have someone drive me to the test?

- How long will the test take?

- Will the test cause pain or discomfort?

- What are the risks and benefits of this test?

- When can I get the results of the test?

This way, you have all the information you need, so you can evaluate with the help of your doctor if a test or procedure is right for you.

Preparation for Tests and Procedures

If you are to have a test or procedure, be sure to follow the instructions given to you by your medical professional in regard to dietary restrictions, medications, and other preparations. Many patients who arrive for a test or procedure haven't followed the preparation instructions and the test has to be canceled or rescheduled.

"My niece had a procedure last week. She was having a growth removed from her lip. She never asked her doctor if she could drive home after the procedure or if she could go back to work the same day. She never asked the price—he wasn't a provider for her insurance.

I talked to her the night before her procedure. She told me she was driving herself to the doctor and she lived forty-five minutes away. She planned on going back to work right after the procedure, a thirty-minute drive.

I told her to call the doctor at 8 AM when they opened and ask what pain meds (if any) she'd be on and if she could drive, go to work, drive home after work, etc. She didn't call the doctor the morning of her procedure. Her appointment was at 10 AM.

After her minor surgical procedure, she was in a lot of pain when the anesthetic wore off. She drove to my house—she was too miserable to even fill her prescription. I gave her an ice pack (which was part of the post-op instructions) and drove to get her prescription filled. She stayed with me all day. By 8 PM she was feeling well enough to drive home."

Anonymous Aunt of the Patient, Atlanta, GA

Follow Up on Test Results

If you undergo tests, it is imperative that you follow up with the doctor who ordered the test and ask for the results. No news is not necessarily good news. Doctors and their staff get busy and might not call you with your results.

Ask for copies of the results and place them in your health file. Discuss the results with your doctor.

Request that your test results also be sent to your PCP and any other specialist involved in your care.

Tests and the Practice of Defensive Medicine

Defensive medicine is defined as medical practices created to prevent the possibility of malpractice lawsuits. It is the fear of getting sued that makes some doctors order more tests to protect themselves rather than putting their patients' needs first.

Physicians are in a difficult position. Our legal system is set up to encourage defensive medicine. A study published in the *Archives of Internal Medicine* (June 28, 2010) reported that 90.7 percent of doctors believe that protections against malpractice suits are needed in order to decrease the ordering of unnecessary medical tests. Ask questions about the tests that your doctors order.

The other side of this issue is that no patient wants her doctor to miss anything. Just know that it is possible that some doctors may order more tests than are medically necessary.

Surgeries

If your doctor recommends surgery, ask questions. Before you agree to surgery, you must understand what the surgery is, what the limitations are, what the risks are, what surgery can and cannot do and how long the recovery period will be. You will want to ask the surgeon for the anticipated results of the surgery.

Create a list of questions before you meet with the surgeon and bring your medical journal with you so you can write down the answers and refer to them later.

It is helpful to discuss the information about your proposed surgery with a trusted loved one, in particular one who is medically savvy. If you have a family member who is a physician, discuss the surgery with her as well. Discuss the possibility of surgery with your PCP.

"Patients that have acute gallbladder attacks or a hernia that don't have the necessary medical intervention/surgery, will continue to have problems. They may be traveling when their condition worsens and will then be forced to have surgery and may have to go to a mediocre hospital and not have the surgeon of their choice. By not taking care of the problem proactively and waiting until their condition becomes acute, they may need a more complicated surgery. Don't be in denial. Don't say it won't happen to you."

Rafael Reisfeld, MD, General Surgery, Los Angeles, CA

Sample questions for your surgeon:

- What is the name of the surgery you want to perform?

- Is your fee covered by my health insurance?

- Is the hospital or surgery center covered by my health insurance?

- Is the anesthesiologist's fee covered by my insurance?
- Do you have informational materials you can give me about this type of surgery?
- How many of these surgeries have you performed? What is your success rate?
- Would you mind if I talk to one or two of your other patients who had this surgery?
- What will the surgery do for me?
- What happens if the surgery is not successful?
- What are the risks of this type of surgery?
- Will the surgery be performed in the hospital or in a surgery center?
- What will my recovery be like? (How long will it take? How active can I be? What restrictions will I have?)
- Will I be in pain after the surgery?
- Will I need someone to help with my care after the surgery?
- What will happen if I don't have this surgery?

Understand Informed Consent

Informed consent means that you know how your illness or condition will be treated. It also means you agree to the operation or treatment. You will be asked to sign paperwork. If you do not understand any aspect of your surgery, ask questions.

Get a Second Opinion

If you have been told you need surgery, get a second opinion. Even if you have full confidence in this surgeon, get a second opinion. You may find out that the first surgeon was correct, but you may also find that there are alternatives to surgery. You also might find out more information about the surgery that will benefit you in your aftercare.

It might be tempting to jump into surgery if you are in severe pain or if you are fearful about your medical condition. Both are understandable motivations for rushing into surgery, but unless it is an emergency, try to wait until you have had time to process the idea of having surgery, get a second opinion, research your surgeon and more.

"I know a patient who went to see a doctor she'd seen for knee problems because she'd recently developed back pain. Her doctor asked her to have an MRI of her spine. The MRI showed arthritis in her lower back. He walked her across the hall to another orthopedist's office, a spine surgeon. After looking at the patient's MRI, the spine surgeon told her she needed an urgent, complex back operation. The patient listened to the spine surgeon and ten days later proceeded with a surgery that left her partially paralyzed and in a wheelchair for the rest of her life.

She should first have been provided with physical therapy or offered a simple back operation with minimal complexity. This is one example of how patients will go to specialists and feel obligated to follow that doctor's advice."

Anonymous MD, UCLA David Geffen School of Medicine,
Los Angeles, CA

Ask About Alternatives to Surgery

Ask the surgeon if there are any alternatives to surgery.

Several surgeons I interviewed said that patients sometimes think that surgery is the answer. Each of them said that it isn't always the answer. Ask your surgeon what your options are. You might be tempted to leap into surgery with the first surgeon you meet. Maybe you're in a lot of pain or maybe you have a serious disease and you want it taken care of. This is very understandable. But you can't turn back the clock after surgery. Do your homework before you agree to it.

Be Aware of Money-Driven Surgeries, Tests and Treatments

A physician at a highly respected medical institution said, "Patients should always understand that there can be a financial motivation to do tests, treatments and surgeries. In the private sector, the incentive is to do more tests and treatments. In managed care, the incentive is to do less."

Research Your Surgeon

Make sure your surgeon is board certified and affiliated with your hospital of choice.

Many people choose their surgeon based on word of mouth and how comfortable they feel with her, but it's equally important to examine the doctor's credentials. Check state disciplinary records. Every state has a database of licensed physicians and any disciplinary actions against them.

You can't unring the bell once surgery has been performed. It's well worth it to research ahead of time. Please don't blindly trust any doctor or any surgeon. There are plenty of very qualified surgeons out there—you want to make sure you have one of them.

Your medical care is a team sport. Do your part and participate. Here's how:

- Go to the surgeon's website, if she has one. Look up her bio or CV. Check board certification, hospitals she is affiliated with and any specialties she is certified in. Make sure you are comfortable with all the information you find. It is a good sign if your surgeon is affiliated with a highly respected medical school.

- If the surgeon does not have a website, call her office and ask that her bio or CV be emailed, faxed or mailed to you.

- Remember the question about asking your surgeon if you can speak to one or two of her patients who have had the same surgery you are considering? Call those patients now. Ask them how they like the surgeon, if the surgery was successful, and if they were satisfied with the care they received from this surgeon.

Research the Surgery Center or Hospital

Consider researching the hospital or surgery center ahead of time.

If you have to stay in the hospital as an inpatient, research that hospital for patient safety indicators, top ten procedures performed, accreditation by a national accrediting organization and quality awards and ratings.

According to the American Cancer Society, the best hospitals offer pathology labs, diagnostic labs, blood banks, around-the-clock staffing, social work services and intensive care units.

Discuss the Surgery with Your Primary Care Physician

Part of your PCP's job is to be "captain of the ship" when it comes to your medical care. Discuss this surgery with your PCP and ask all the necessary questions. Ask this doctor's opinion of the surgeon. Ask how you can find out more information about this surgeon and the surgery itself.

I was to have minor surgery in a surgery center. I met with my internist to discuss it. I brought in all of my pertinent medical records, asked him to review them, asked questions, and then asked his opinion about it. I wanted a second set of eyes and ears involved in my medical care in this situation. Once I had his blessing, I felt confident to go forward with the surgery.

Tips for Scheduling Surgery

- Try not to schedule your surgery on the Friday before a holiday weekend. Doctors can be away that weekend and you want your surgeon around, not a doctor on call who does not know you, in case there is a problem. If you are recovering in a hospital, holiday weekends are notorious for reduced nursing staff, meaning that each nurse can be responsible for more patients. This can lead to a higher probability of medical error.

- Try to schedule your surgery as the first or second one of the day. Your surgeon will have a lot more energy first thing in the morning than later on in the day.

- If you are having surgery in a teaching hospital, try to avoid scheduling in July, when new interns are starting out in the hospital. More medical errors occur at this time.

Learn about Your Anesthesia

Find out if the anesthesiologist's fee is covered by your health insurance plan. Even if your doctor takes your insurance, it doesn't always mean the anesthesiologist does. Ask questions. You could end up with a bill after surgery that you didn't expect.

Before your surgery, you will have an opportunity to talk with the anesthesiologist. If you have any concerns or previous reactions to anesthesia, this is the time to discuss them.

Schedule a Follow-Up Appointment with the Surgeon

You must see the surgeon for a follow-up appointment. She will want to evaluate how you are doing. This is very important.

> *"I know of a nurse who went to a cardiac surgeon. After her surgery, she saw the physician's assistant, not the surgeon. After I've done surgery on a patient, I want to make sure you're okay. I want to shake your hand."*
>
> Charles A. Hunter, MD, FACS, General Surgery, Los Angeles, CA

Seeing the surgeon who did your surgery is very important not only because she saw you and evaluated your medical condition before the surgery, but also because she'll want to know if things are going as planned with your recovery.

> *"A patient had blood in his urine. He had managed care insurance. He went to his PCP and got an urgent referral to a kidney specialist. The patient had testing that revealed kidney cancer. The patient had surgery to remove his kidney. The kidney doctor never told the patient to return for a follow up. The patient never saw the kidney doctor for a follow up visit. He did not go for a check up or annual physical with his PCP.*
>
> *The patient wasn't feeling well a year later and he went to see his PCP. This doctor sent him for a follow-up kidney x-ray. The radiologist who was doing his kidney x-ray suggested a chest x-ray as well. The chest x-ray revealed that the kidney cancer had metastasized to the patient's lung.*
>
> *This patient was in his early forties and died less than a year later after many rounds of chemotherapy."*
>
> Rae, Registered Nurse, Beverly Hills, CA

PATIENT CHECKLIST

- ☐ Do I need any screening tests?

- ☐ If I need a test, do I fully understand what it is, what the doctor is looking for and why I need to have it?

- ☐ Have I asked if there are any risks or side effects?

- ☐ Do I understand how to prepare for a test, procedure or surgery?

- ☐ Can I drive home afterward?

- ☐ Does my insurance cover the test or procedure?

- ☐ If I need surgery, did I ask for the name of the surgery and what it is for?

- ☐ Are there alternatives to surgery?

- ☐ What will happen if I don't have the surgery?

- ☐ Did I talk to my primary care physician about the surgery?

- ☐ What will the recovery time be?

- ☐ Will I need help at home during my recovery?

- ☐ What are the benefits and risks of the surgery?

- ☐ Did I research the surgeon carefully?

- ☐ Did I research the hospital or surgery center?

- ☐ Does my health insurance cover the surgery and the hospital or surgery center?

- ☐ Do I need a second opinion?

18

The Hospital

*"Despite the best of intentions, you cannot rely
on the hospital staff to protect you against day-to-day/
run-of-the-mill mistakes. You want to trust everyone—
especially in that environment—but you can't."*

MICHAEL A. WEISS, AUTHOR,
PATIENT ADVOCATE, WEST ORANGE, NJ

A few years ago I wrote *Critical Conditions: The Essential Hospital Guide To Get Your Loved One Out Alive.* I highly recommend it if you or a loved one will be hospitalized. It contains much more information about how to have a successful and safe hospital stay than will fit in this chapter.

You might think that hospitals are the safest places to be if you are sick, injured or seriously ill. In many cases they are. However, there are some sobering statistics about hospital patient deaths caused by preventable medical errors. Nearly a quarter of a million deaths in hospitals nationwide were found to be preventable (the Sixth Annual HealthGrades Patient Safety in American Hospitals Study, 2010).

That certainly doesn't make any of us feel any better. But as a take-charge patient, there is plenty you can do to keep yourself safe in the hospital. Do a little preparation before you go, read the information below and remember your single most valuable asset in the hospital—your advocate.

Hospitals are completely foreign to most of us. If you have the opportunity to educate yourself before you enter the hospital, you'll be doing yourself a great service. Preparing ahead of time is part of being a take-charge patient. After reading this chapter, you can implement some effective strategies to make your stay as pleasant and safe as possible.

If You're Admitted as a Patient, Get an Advocate

Enlist the help of a loved one to oversee and monitor your care while you are in the hospital. Ask your advocate to bring a notebook in which she will record your medications, diagnoses, tests, procedures, surgeries and daily progress. Your advocate will be your second set of eyes and ears, your watchdog and your support.

Your advocate will also note names and contact information of your primary nurses and physicians. Request that she write down what doctors and nurses say about your condition and treatment plan. If she is unable to be with you most of the time, ask her to enlist two to three other loved ones to take shifts at your bedside. All members of the advocate team will share tasks.

Bring Copies of Your Medical Records to the Hospital

Bring copies of your pertinent medical records, a list of your current medications and their dosages, over-the-counter medications, herbs and supplements and allergies to medications to the hospital. Include a list of any diagnoses your doctors have given you. You want the hospital medical staff to know as much about you as possible.

If you are unable to complete any of these tasks, ask your advocate to do it for you.

Create a Patient Safety Checklist

Create your own patient safety checklist. Recite this checklist to each new medical professional you encounter. This is a very effective way to prevent certain medical errors.

When you encounter any new medical professional, recite the following information:

- Your full name
- Your date of birth

- Your physician's name

- The test or procedure you are supposed to have

- If you are to have surgery, recite the type of surgery and the site on your body to be operated on. Mark the spot on your body with a permanent marker

- Show your hospital wrist band to every medical professional you encounter

If you are shy about verbally repeating a checklist to medical professionals, you can ask politely like this: "Would you mind if I go over a few things before we begin? I'm not doubting you, I just want to play a role in my safety."

I created a patient safety checklist for patients and their advocates to use in the hospital to prevent fatal medical errors. Go to www.CriticalConditions .com to download a free copy.

Prevent Medication Errors

Approximately 1.5 million people are injured by medication errors every year. No one is trying to make mistakes. Medication names can look alike and sound alike, prescriptions may be unreadable or written illegibly or scanned or input into the computer improperly.

To prevent being given the wrong medication or dosage, you are simply going to double-check every medication you are given in the hospital to make sure you don't get the wrong one. If you are not up to this task, ask your advocate to help.

Create a list of all the medications you are taking. This includes new medications prescribed for you since your admission to the hospital. Write down the name of each medication (both brand and generic), the dosage, how often you are supposed to take it, a description of the medication and the label and what the medication is for. If you are unable to complete this task, ask your advocate to do it for you.

Each time you are to be given a medication, ask for the name of the medication, the dosage and what it is for. If you are given medication from an IV bag, note the name and how the label appears. If something looks new or different, ask questions. Perhaps you can say, "Would you mind telling me what these medications are? I just want to take part in my medical care. Thank you."

Be sure you know what medication you are being given and the correct dosage. If you don't understand why you are taking a certain medication or what it is for, ask questions. Speak up.

Establish a Relationship with Your Primary Nurse

Your primary nurse is the registered nurse who is responsible for your daily care. Besides the doctor, she is the only medical professional in the hospital who can give you medication and respond to your pain management needs.

Hospital staff dress alike so make sure you know which one is your primary nurse. You will have two primary nurses every day—one for the morning and one for the evening. Get personal. Show appreciation to your primary nurses. Most primary nurses are saints so a little goodwill from you goes a long way. The more gratitude you express to these professionals, the more attention you will receive. And more attention translates to the probability of fewer errors. Have a loved one bring you a few thank-you cards. Address them to your primary nurses with a few words about how much you appreciate their good care.

Your advocate can ask if she may assist with your care. This shows that she is involved. Doctors and nurses all said that if patients have involved family members, they get more attention. More attention leads to better care.

My mother and godmother were patients in the hospital for extended stays, five months and seven months respectively. I learned to ingratiate myself to their nurses by offering to help. I asked what I could do to assist and showed my appreciation by thanking them and by bringing cookies and treats on a regular basis. This led to a friendly relationship. My good relationships with them benefited my mother's and godmother's care.

Meet with Your Doctors

You want face-to-face interaction with your doctors, not only to establish relationships, but to get information about your care directly from them.

Ask your advocate to join you during doctors' rounds so she can take notes on conversations. It's handy to have someone there to ask the questions you may have forgotten. Prepare questions ahead of time about your diagnosis, treatment and prognosis.

Remember to humanize yourself to your physicians. Think about how many patients these medical professionals see in a week. You want each and every one to see you as a human being, not as the "shoulder surgery" in room 209. Create a personal connection.

Ask Questions

Many people are afraid to question their nurses and doctors. Don't be. If a medication looks new or different, ask for its name and what it is for. If something seems amiss or you are surprised by some piece of information, such as orders for discharge when you thought you were going to be in the hospital for another two days, ask questions. As long as you are polite and respectful, your request should be met with respect. If you don't understand something, ask questions. This is your health and well-being we are talking about. Be assertive.

Be Alert on Holidays and Weekends and at Night

Medical errors increase at these times. There are fewer nurses per patient and doctors can be away. Ask your advocate to be with you as much as possible or hire a sitter, companion or private duty nurse to fill in.

Take Action If a Problem Occurs

If there is a problem with a medical professional who is caring for you, ask your advocate to speak to the nurse supervisor or charge nurse about it.

When my godmother was in the hospital for heart surgery, she told me that the nurse who took care of her at night was not nice to her. Martha said that this woman was rough and acted angry. Martha begged me not to tell anyone because she was afraid that word would get back to the nurse and her treatment would worsen. I found the charge nurse and explained the situation. The nurse was removed from Martha's care.

If there is a more serious problem such as a medical error, contact the hospital's ombudsman. This professional functions as a liaison between patients and the hospital system. Part of her job is to find answers to questions and solutions to concerns and grievances that are part of hospitalization. The ombudsman facilitates communication between patients and medical professionals, educates patients and their families, and advocates for patients' rights.

Older Patients

You might think that admitting an older adult to the hospital is as simple as dropping her off at "Admitting" and allowing the hospital staff to take care of the rest. Think again. Older adults desperately need your help because a hospital stay can be fraught with medical errors, medication mistakes, falls, infectious diseases, bedsores and more.

Hospital medical staff want the very best care for your older loved one but they are under tremendous pressure. Few can overcome patient overload, a nationwide nursing shortage and a developing physician shortage. Many hospitals in the United States are unable to accommodate all of the needs and vulnerabilities of older adults.

Your older loved one might need your help getting to the bathroom, eating a meal or asking her primary nurse to come to her room to administer pain medication. If she is bedridden, she may ring the buzzer for the nurse several times without anyone responding. Often, nurses have too many patients to take care of and can't get to each patient right away. If your older loved one is unable to get out of bed, consider being there to lend a hand.

"When my mom was in the hospital recovering from an unplanned hip replacement, I realized how helpful it was for her to have me with her to provide comfort and be her advocate. In the days following her surgery, Mom was in pain, consistently nauseous and exhausted. She did not want to eat or get out of bed and was reluctant to participate in physical therapy. During the week she was in the hospital, I spent the better part of every day at her side. Much of what I did was prodding—whether it was to take a few bites of a meal when she had no appetite, walk from the bed to sit in a chair or practice her leg exercises when all she wanted to do was sleep. It became clear to me that no matter how kind the nurses were, they did not have the time to spend with her to do these things...the very basic things that her

recovery hinged upon, such as getting adequate nutrition and
exercising her brand new hip."

Nancy, Daughter of the Patient, Santa Monica, CA

You as a family member or good friend must monitor an older adult's medical care and provide support during a hospital stay.

"I take care of both my mother and father. They both are
housebound and have multiple medical issues. My father has
the beginning stages of dementia. After taking my father to the
hospital with severe heart pains on several occasions, the doctors
released him each time and sent him home. I was so disgusted
that I removed him from his HMOs and immediately put him on
Medicare/Medi-Cal. I took him to my mother's primary doctor
who referred me to a cardiologist who found my dad had a 100%
blocked artery and two more with 85% blockage. He needed
triple bypass surgery."

Mary J. Avila, Daughter of the Patient, South San Gabriel, CA

Older Patients Are More at Risk

"There was something wrong with my mom, I could tell. She was
not feeling well, and not herself. I took her to the ER and they
didn't find anything. They wanted to send her home. I told the
person on staff that I wasn't comfortable with taking her home.
Meanwhile, I prayed that they would find what was wrong so she
could be treated. Turns out, she had a severe infection and her
organs shut down. They found a stone lodged in her intestines.
What would have happened if I had let the hospital discharge
her? I was persistent."

Mary J. Avila, Daughter of the Patient, South San Gabriel, CA

Delirium occurs in one third of hospitalized patients over the age of sixty-five and in more than 70 percent of older people in intensive care units. Reasons for this include serious illness, exposure to new medications, disruption of normal routines and sleep disturbance. Family members are often the first to notice changes that might indicate delirium.

If an older adult cannot reposition herself, she is at risk for pressure ulcers (bedsores). Pressure ulcers affect 1 million adults annually.

An older patient may have multiple medical issues, requiring several specialists to be involved in her case. This can be confusing and difficult to coordinate for any patient.

New medications may be introduced that can lead to side effects. Older patients may already be taking multiple medications, which can lead to adverse effects.

"I found out that I could be an advocate for Mom when she was too weak to speak up for herself. Between her pain and nausea, she was getting an abundance of medication. Not much seemed to be helping and a lot of it made her too sleepy to get out of bed. I worked out a plan with her doctor and the nurses to give her pain medication half an hour before getting out of bed or starting physical therapy to make her more comfortable and willing to move around. Other medications to relieve anxiety were withheld until bedtime to help her sleep through the night. Changing the medication schedule made Mom more willing to participate in her own recovery, as well as get the rest she desperately needed."

Nancy, Daughter of the Patient, Santa Monica, CA

Older adults are at risk for falls, especially if they are sedated or disoriented. Among older adults, falls are the leading cause of injury and death.

Older adults can be at risk for malnutrition. Studies cite that 58 percent of patients sixty-five and older have problems eating. The nutritional status of older patients has been reported to diminish in hospitals. This can slow recovery.

What You Can Do to Help Your Older Loved One

- Be sure your loved one has her glasses and hearing aids.
- Make your loved one's hospital room feel more like home. Older patients do better in the hospital if some of their routine is maintained and they have some familiar items around. Bring the outside world into the hospital room. This might include a cozy comforter, photos

of family and friends, a clock to keep track of time and her address book should she want to contact loved ones. Books, newspapers, music and videos go a long way.

- If your loved one is unable to reposition herself in bed, monitor how many times her body is turned to prevent pressure ulcers (bedsores). Ask her primary nurse to help you with this.

  My godmother had a bedsore nearly the size of a football on her backside. I reminded the nurses to turn her every two hours. I helped them do it.

- Be aware of behavior and mood changes. In a notebook, document how your loved one is doing on a daily basis. Be aware of any sudden mood or cognitive changes such as drowsiness, apathy, confusion, little or no speech or movement, agitation or hallucinations. If you notice a sudden change, bring it to the attention of her physician and primary nurse. Ask for an evaluation.

- Monitor your loved one's meals. Sometimes older patients have a difficult time eating and may need some assistance. Sometimes the meal tray is taken away before the patient has had a chance to eat. Monitor dietary restrictions to make sure she receives meals the doctor has ordered. You can also bring in meals from home, but check with the patient's primary nurse first.

- If your loved one is at risk of falling, be present at her bedside at all times. Ask family or friends to help you by taking shifts. You can also hire a sitter or private duty nurse to assist. This prevents the need for restraints. Although restraints are for patient safety, they often add to the patient's confusion and increase agitation and fear.

- Last but not least, provide comfort to the patient. She may be frightened in the hospital and may feel even more uncomfortable with her loss of control than you do. Reassure her that you are watching out for her.

Resources to Research Hospitals

- The Joint Commission
  http://jointcommission.org/

- HealthGrades
  http://healthgrades.com/

- Hospital Compare
  http://hospitalcompare.hhs.gov/

- The Leapfrog Group
  http://Leapfroggroup.org/

PATIENT SAFETY CHECKLIST

☐   Do I have an advocate?

☐   Do I have my patient safety checklist?

☐   Did I create my list of medications, their dosages, over-the-counter medications, herbs and supplements? Have I included my allergies to medications?

☐   Did I list new medications the doctors prescribed?

☐   Do I know who my primary nurses are? Have I written down their names?

☐   Is my advocate willing to be with me during doctors' rounds?

☐   Did I create a list of questions for the doctors and primary nurses?

☐   Did I get extra help for weekends, nights and holidays?

☐   Do I have a notebook for me and my advocate to take notes in?

☐   Do I understand my diagnosis and treatment plan?

19

Urgent Care Centers, Retail Medical Clinics and the Emergency Room

"Urgent care centers are not all created equal. Try to find one that is affiliated with a primary practice."

NONA L. HANSON, MD, FAMILY MEDICINE, OCEANSIDE, CA

If you aren't aware that medical care is offered outside of your primary care physician's office, you are not alone. Years ago, I did not know what an urgent care center was until a family member was in need and her doctor's office was closed for the day. I also did not know that many pharmacies now have retail medical clinics.

Urgent care does not replace your primary care physician. An urgent care center is a convenient option when your regular physician is away or when medical care is needed outside of regular office hours. Urgent care centers and retail medical clinics can be less expensive than a doctor visit or a visit to the emergency room at a hospital. As a take-charge patient, you will have to find out about fees.

Please remember that if you have a serious medical condition or injury, call your primary care physician right away or go to your nearest emergency room.

Urgent Care Centers

An estimated 17 percent of all patients who visit U.S. hospital emergency departments could be treated at urgent care centers or retail medical clinics instead, a move that would save $4.4 billion a year in health care costs, a new U.S. study suggests. Lacerations, sprains and minor infections are among the conditions that can be treated safely outside of hospitals, according to a RAND Corporation study published in the October 2010 issue of the journal *Health Affairs*.

Urgent care centers are open during the day, in the evenings and on weekends, and allow for walk-in appointments. They offer you a place to go for medical treatment outside of the emergency room of a hospital if your primary care physician's office is closed. Urgent care centers are used to treat patients who have an injury or illness that requires immediate attention but is not serious enough to warrant a trip to the ER.

Physicians and nurses are on staff at urgent care centers.

Common Medical Conditions Treated at Urgent Care Centers

- Ear infections
- Sprains
- Urinary tract infections
- Vomiting
- High fevers
- Coughs, colds, sore throats
- Skin rashes
- Fevers or flu
- Wounds
- Animal bites
- Mild asthma

Most urgent care centers also offer immunizations, school and athletic physicals and health exams for men and women. Many have on-site pharmacies.

Tips to Find a Good Urgent Care Center

- If you have a primary care physician or pediatrician, ask if her practice is affiliated with an urgent care center. If it's after hours, you can always call the physician's answering service and ask the same question.

- Ask friends and family which urgent care centers they have had good experiences with.

- Ask your doctor if she can recommend a good urgent care center if she is not affiliated with one. Place this information in your health file.

Benefits of Urgent Care Centers

Urgent care centers can be more cost effective than the emergency room at a hospital for the conditions listed above, but you will have to ask about costs. In addition, wait time in urgent care centers is usually shorter than in the ER. Health insurance plans might pay a higher benefit for urgent care centers than for ER visits. If you need to go to an urgent care center, try to find one that takes your insurance. Call ahead and ask questions.

Retail Medical Clinics (Minute Clinics, Take Care, MediMinute)

A convenient option for people seeking routine care without visiting the doctor's office or a hospital ER is a retail medical clinic.

These clinics are located in some Walgreens, CVS pharmacies, other pharmacies and some supermarkets. AeroClinic operates out of some airports.

Some doctors said that retail medical clinics have their place. They're great for routine vaccinations such as annual flu shots. They unclog PCP offices.

Nearly all retail medical clinics accept insurance plans, and they are usually attached to pharmacies. They are staffed with nurse practitioners or physician's assistants and many offer wellness and preventative services, physical exams and vaccinations.

Common Conditions Treated at Retail Medical Clinics

- Minor illnesses

- Minor injuries

- Allergic reactions

- Urinary tract infections

- Upper respiratory infections

- Sinusitis

- Strep throat

- Flu

- Animal bites

- Conjunctivitis

Come Prepared When You Visit Urgent Care Centers and Retail Medical Clinics

- Bring your health summary with a list of current medications and dosages and allergies to medications, medical conditions, recent surgeries or procedures, plus the name and contact information of your primary care doctor.

- Ask for a copy of your record from the visit and give it to your primary care physician. Even if you request that an urgent care center or retail medical clinic send your records to your PCP, it may not happen. If you request your own copy at the time of service you won't have a gap in your medical records. For example, you may need a record of the antibiotic or immunization you received.

"Retail medical clinics are great. Patients can avoid the ER or urgent care. There is a shorter wait time, and patients can often spend more time with the nurse practitioner. It is important to have medical history, a list of medications/herbal supplements, and allergies to food and medications, so there are no gaps and patients will receive proper care."

Karen Rozdal, RN, BSN, Huntington Beach, CA

Hospital Emergency Rooms (ERs)

If you have an emergency, call your PCP first and ask if you should visit the emergency room of a hospital. ERs specialize in acute care. You do not need an appointment to be seen at an ER.

The ER provides initial treatment for a broad spectrum of illnesses and injuries, some of which may be life threatening and may require immediate attention.

The ER departments of most hospitals are open twenty-four hours a day and are staffed by nurses, doctors and other medical professionals.

You should go to the ER if you have any of the following medical issues. This is not an all-inclusive list and not a recommendation of any kind. You must use your own judgment.

- Chest pain
- Shortness of breath
- Severe abdominal pain following an injury
- Uncontrolled bleeding
- Confusion or loss of consciousness
- Poisoning or suspected poisoning
- Serious burns, cuts or infections
- Inability to swallow
- Seizures
- Paralysis
- Broken bones
- Other serious injuries

PATIENT CHECKLIST

☐ Do I understand my options if I need medical care after hours or on weekends?

☐ Do I understand when I should go to an urgent care center, retail medical clinic or the ER of a hospital?

20

Prevention—Your Health

*"It's always easier to prevent a disease
rather than treat it."*

JOYCE RUBIN, MD, INTERNAL MEDICINE,
PENNSYLVANIA HOSPITAL, PHILADELPHIA, PA

P art of being proactive with your health is prevention. Taking care of
yourself might not seem like a top priority when you're younger, but if
you develop an illness, you'll wish you'd done it sooner. None of us really
wants to ask any of these questions or do any of these screenings, but think
of it this way—it's so much easier to have annual physicals, get screenings,
and ask questions about your health problems now rather than wait until you
think something is seriously wrong. At that point, you may have to do more.

General Health Tips for Women

This is our health we are talking about. When we were twenty years
old, we thought nothing would ever happen to us and believed we were
superhuman. As we get older, we realize that if we don't have our health,
we have nothing. As a take-charge patient, make health your number one
priority. I interviewed female OB/GYNs and internists who said that women
put their health last, that their health comes after dealing with their families,
their jobs and their homes.

It's time to value your health, get proactive about it and realize that
putting your health last leaves you at a disadvantage.

"Women put themselves second. They're the primary caretakers most of the time. They take care of the kids, the house, the husband, and more. Mothers feel guilty about putting themselves first. It's important to realize that you're going to be at your best if you're taking care of yourself."

Alison Garb, MD, Internal Medicine, Pacific Palisades, CA

- Get an annual physical checkup.

- Get the screenings you need. Ask your physician about screenings and tests that look for diseases before you have symptoms. Keep in mind that when dealing with a disease it is always easier to treat earlier rather than later.

- If your doctor recommends a procedure for you, ask questions, do your research and then make the appointment and get it done. Most of us do not want to undergo exploratory procedures, but take-charge patients have them anyway to prevent serious disease.

Breast Cancer

Ask your doctor, nurse practitioner or physician's assistant when a mammogram is right for you. This decision should take into account your age, family history, overall health and personal concerns.

If you have concerns about breast cancer or if breast cancer runs in your family, you might consider discussing BRCA testing with your physician.

The BRCA Test

The BRCA test is a blood test to check for specific changes (mutations) in genes that help control normal cell growth. Finding changes in these genes, called BRCA1 and BRCA2, can help determine your chance of developing breast cancer or ovarian cancer. Genetic counseling before and after a BRCA test is very important to help you understand the benefits, risks and possible outcomes of the test. A BRCA gene test does not test for cancer itself. This test is only done for people with a strong family history of breast cancer or ovarian cancer, and sometimes for those who already have one of these diseases.

Cervical Cancer

The Department of Health and Human Services recommends that you have a Pap smear every one to three years if you are between the ages of twenty-one and sixty-five and have been sexually active.

Sexually Transmitted Diseases

Ask your doctor if you should be screened for sexually transmitted diseases such as chlamydia.

General Health Tips for Men

Several doctors said that many men are not proactive about their health. These medical professionals said that it's your significant others who get you in to see your doctors. Part of being a take-charge patient is being responsible for your health. If your doctor recommends getting an annual checkup and screenings, try not to wait until the loved ones in your life push you to do it.

> "You come to the realization that preventative medicine is a whole lot better than reactive medicine—less expensive, less risk. The longer you wait, the more risk you have to accept."
>
> Thomas C. Fisher, Patient, Naples, FL

It's easy to deny health problems and avoid the doctor. Consider taking charge of yourself as a patient and making that appointment with your doctor or other medical professional before you are urged to do so by others.

Abdominal Aortic Aneurysm

The U.S. Department of Health and Human Services recommends that if you are between the ages of sixty-five and seventy-five, you should talk to your doctor or other medical professional about being screened for an abdominal aortic aneurism. If someone in your immediate family has an aortic aneurism, ask your doctor or other medical professional if you should be checked.

Prostate Cancer Screening

Professional organizations vary in their recommendations about who should or should not have a PSA screening for prostate cancer. Organizations that do recommend a PSA screening encourage men to get the test when they are between the ages of forty and seventy-five or have an increased risk of prostate cancer. Discuss this with your doctor or other medical professional.

Sexually Transmitted Diseases
Ask your doctor if you should be screened for sexually transmitted diseases such as syphilis.

General Tips for Men and Women

Colorectal Cancer
Starting at age fifty, it is recommended that you have a screening test for colorectal cancer. If you have a family history of this type of cancer, you may need to be screened earlier. Ask your doctor.

> "I have a female patient who I've seen for 15 years. Starting at the age of 50, I told her she needed a colonoscopy. She didn't want to do it—she was afraid. She put it off until age 60. She had one and colon cancer was found. She said to me, 'I wish I'd listened to you 10 years ago when you told me.'"
>
> Sheryl A. Ross, MD, Obstetrics and Gynecology,
> Santa Monica, CA

Depression
Your emotional health is just as important as your physical health. Talk to your doctor or other medical professional if you think you might be depressed. Most people have felt sad or low at times. Feeling depressed can be a normal reaction to loss, life's challenges or injured self-esteem.

According to the National Institute of Mental Health, signs and symptoms of depression include

- persistent sad, anxious or "empty" feelings;
- feelings of hopelessness of pessimism;
- feelings of guilt, worthlessness, or helplessness;
- irritability or restlessness;
- loss of interest in activities that once brought you pleasure;
- and more.

Ask your doctor or other medical professional about being screened for depression if you are experiencing any of the above symptoms.

Diabetes

Ask your doctor or other medical professional if you should be screened for diabetes.

High Blood Pressure

If you are eighteen years or older, you should have your blood pressure checked every two years. High blood pressure can cause heart attacks, strokes, kidney and eye problems, and heart failure. Ask your doctor or other medical professional if you need your blood pressure checked.

High Cholesterol

> *"My father had two heart attacks and diabetes. He wouldn't stop smoking and ate a diet high in fat and sugar. He never exercised. My brother and I are doctors. We begged him to eat healthy, exercise, and stop smoking. He refused to heed anyone's advice. He died at 59 of metastatic lung cancer."*
>
> Bernard P. Ginsberg, MD, Family Medicine, Tavernier, FL

According to the U.S. Department of Health and Human Services, if you are twenty years of age or older, you should have your cholesterol checked regularly if

- you use tobacco;
- you are obese;
- you have diabetes or high blood pressure;
- you have a personal history of heart disease or blocked arteries;
- someone in your family had a heart attack before the age of sixty.

HIV

According to the U.S. Department of Health and Human Services, you should talk with your doctor or other medical professionals about an HIV screening if

- you've had unprotected sex with multiple partners;
- you have injected drugs;
- you have or do exchange sex for money or drugs or have sex partners who do;

- you've had a sex partner who is HIV-infected, bisexual or injects drugs;
- you are being treated for a sexually transmitted disease;
- you had a blood transfusion between 1978 and 1985.

Osteoporosis

Doctors recommend that you have a bone density test if you are sixty-five years of age or older. This test checks to see if your bones are strong.

Osteoporosis develops less often in men than in women but in the past few years the problem of osteoporosis in men has been recognized as an important public health issue, particularly in men over the age of seventy.

Talk to your doctor or other medical professional about when you should have this test.

Overweight and Obesity

Talk to your doctor or other medical professional about whether you are overweight. If you are, you can ask for help with diet, exercise tips and strategies.

"I had a patient who was overweight. He was an ex-police officer, inactive, with diabetes and high blood pressure. I knew any day there was a possibility that he could have a heart attack or stroke. He didn't want to know about medications or about his diabetes. One day, it clicked. He started going to diabetes clinics I sent him to. He started to keep track of his food intake. He lost sixty pounds and he is off all of his medications. He took a vested interest in his health. Between my communication with him and other resources, he took a vested interest in his own body. I love that. He is my star patient."

Linda Nadwodny, DO, FAAFP, Family Medicine, Lansdale, PA

Immunizations

Vaccines fuel much debate. As a take-charge patient, educate yourself about the risks and benefits of vaccinations and then decide if they are right for you. Some people need vaccinations because they never got them as children. If you did get childhood immunizations, you must ask your doctor or other medical professional if you need them repeated, as some vaccines don't last for a lifetime. As you age, you become more susceptible to infection. More than 50,000 adults in the United States die annually from vaccine-preventable diseases. Ask your doctor which vaccines you should have and when.

You may see several doctors over your lifetime, making it difficult for them to keep track of your vaccines. This is where you come in. Keep track.

Resources

- U.S. Department of Health and Human Services
  http://www.healthfinder.gov

- Medline Plus—A Service of the U.S. National Library of Medicine
  National Institute of Health
  http://www.nlm.nih.gov/medlineplus/

- Centers for Disease Control and Prevention
  http://www.cdc.gov/

- National Institute of Mental Health
  http://www.nimh.nih.gov/health/publications/depression/
  what-is-depression.shtml

PATIENT CHECKLIST

☐ Have I scheduled an appointment for a yearly checkup with my doctor?

☐ Have I asked my doctors about any screenings I need?

☐ Have I had my blood pressure checked recently?

☐ Did I ask my doctor about any immunizations I need?

21

Religious Professionals
and How They Can Help You

"I act as an advocate. There are times
when there is no one around and the patient is alone.
Sometimes I talk to the nurses and hospital chaplain
about the patient's needs and act as an advocate
for that patient."

RABBI MORLEY T. FEINSTEIN, MAHL, MAHE, DD, LOS ANGELES, CA

SPECIAL NOTE: I did not purposely leave out specific religious institutions in this chapter. There is only room for so much. If you have a religious affiliation that is not mentioned here, please go to your place of worship and ask about what they offer to help patients. This is a very brief overview of what churches, synagogues and other religious institutions offer to those in need of care and advocacy.

Before I wrote this book, I had no idea that religious institutions offered so much help to those in need. When I was sick for sixteen months with my medical condition, I consistently called the prayer line of our church to ask for prayers for an accurate diagnosis, treatment plan and the best doctor to help me.

When I was about to have surgery I again called the prayer line. The woman I'd spoken to several times in the past asked, "You're still dealing with this medical condition and pain?" I told her that I was. I also explained that I was going in for surgery and I needed prayer for it to be successful. She put me on the prayer chain.

Soon after, I received a call from our minister and the associate minister asking if I would like to be visited in the hospital and prayed with before my surgery. I received flowers from the church deacons and cards and meals from church friends. I was very touched by everyone's support.

Many religious institutions, such as churches, synagogues and others, offer help to members and nonmembers who are in need. Faith communities can provide much needed support if you are ill, have a serious medical condition, are in the hospital, need to have surgery, are elderly or are homebound. If you are living apart from family and face medical challenges, by all means go to your religious institution and ask for help. Even if you have family and friends close by, sometimes there is no replacement for a spiritual advisor in a time of need.

If You Are Sick

One of the main goals of churches, synagogues and other religious institutions is to help those who are ill and in need. The bigger the religious institution, the more resources they might have. How those resources are allocated varies by religious institution.

> "Let your pastor know if you are scheduled for surgery, are in the hospital, or if you have a medical condition. Some assume the pastor will know."
>
> William H. Craig, DMin,
> Pasadena, CA

If you are a member of a faith community, contact your minister, rabbi, deacon or other religious leader and find out what they offer to those in need. Get involved and ask questions.

Faith communities do so much good. Offering help to those in need is a principle that a number of them are based on.

If you belong to a faith community, don't be shy about asking for help. That is what they are there for.

If You Are in the Hospital

Several religious professionals I spoke to said that just the presence of a minister, rabbi or other faith community leader in the hospital room with a patient improves the quality of care. One minister said that when he visits patients, he creates an additional level of respect for the patient when the patient interacts with doctors, nurses and other medical professionals.

"As a rule, I make the first visit to a patient either at their home or in the hospital. I assess the patient's needs and set up a system of visitors or I continue to go myself."

Rabbi Baruch Hect,
Los Angeles, CA

"The presence of a minister in a hospital room with the patient results in better service. One eighty-two-year-old lady fractured her hip. She went to the hospital. They recommended surgery and another hip replacement. She was frail. One of our church members went with her to the hospital, was with her through the process. This lady got the best service because she had someone with her. Someone else was taking the pressure—helping her to make informed decisions."

Warren G. Booker Jr, DMin, Lexington, MI

If you or a family member is ill or in the hospital, and you would like your rabbi, minister, deacon or other religious professional to visit, you must let them know. Because of HIPAA laws, hospitals are prevented from alerting your faith community if you are a patient there. It is your responsibility to speak up and reach out or ask a loved one to do it for you.

If You Have a Relationship with a Religious Professional
If you have an existing relationship with a religious professional, you can let her know that you are in the hospital and ask her to visit you. According to several ministers, rabbis and other religious professionals, most faith communities have a team or group that helps out their members and even nonmembers who are in the hospital. This may include visitors, and get-well wishes.

In addition to visiting you, your rabbi, minister or other religious professional may interact with the hospital clergy on your behalf regarding observance of religious holidays and rituals. Be sure you or a loved one calls your religious leader and explains your situation so your needs can be met.

Several ministers and rabbis said it is their business to make sure that a patient has visitors from the congregation every day. From daily telephone calls to in-person visits, many faith communities focus on making sure people in need do not feel alone.

> *"When I went into the hospital for serious cardiac surgery, the knowledge that my church was supporting me through an active prayer chain and requested prayers during worship gave me added strength and comfort. But beyond that spiritual element, the ministerial staff visited me in the ICU both pre and post op to offer comfort and prayer. All three of our pastoral staff visited me in the hospital and two at home during recovery. Our then acting head of staff held my hands and prayed with me the night before the surgery. I felt not only a great calmness about the operation ahead, but was convinced that my survival was assured. In addition, congregants who had had similar surgery visited me and called to reassure me that all was going to be well."*

Harvey Mednick, Patient, Los Angeles, CA

If You Don't Have a Relationship with a Religious Professional

If you do not have a preexisting relationship with a religious professional, you can call on the hospital chaplain. Chaplains offer emotional and spiritual support regardless of your denomination. They provide comfort for patients and offer a compassionate ear. Chaplains pray with patients and assist them and their families in making difficult decisions about end-of-life care.

According to a recent *Wall Street Journal* article, hospital chaplains are taking on bigger roles in patient care and are now being integrated into medical teams. Interest in the links between religion, spirituality and health, has given rise to research on how spiritual guidance and discussion can help improve a patient's medical outcome.

A hospital chaplain can also be very helpful if you are from out of town and visiting a hospitalized loved one. When my mother was in the hospital for five months in another state, sometimes the stress and worry over her precarious medical condition really got to me. A nurse I had developed a friendship with suggested that I see the deacon in the hospital. I mentioned that I was not Catholic. She reassured me that hospital chaplains offer nondenominational emotional and spiritual support. I was surprised that this was available. I visited that deacon a number of times while my mother was a patient in the hospital. His support helped ease a very stressful situation.

If You Are Recovering at Home

If you are homebound while recovering from surgery or a hospital stay, your faith community may be able to arrange delivery of meals, assistance with driving to doctor's appointments, help with marketing, etc. Each religious institution will have its own guidelines concerning its services.

> "I recently had surgery and was on bed rest for five weeks. My women's group at my church brought meals to our family for two months. That's a circle of only eight women."
>
> Jackie Koob, RN, Stanton, CA

The thought of coming home from the hospital with no staff to help you can be frightening. Call your faith community and ask for help. You may be bedridden and have visits from home health nurses but sometimes nothing can replace the security of having people visit or call who know you and care about you.

> "Upon my return home after a ten-day hospital stay, a group of church members brought me a homemade lunch every day for two weeks inasmuch as my wife had to go to her office during that time. I also received at least one hundred get-well cards and calls wishing me well. Other members of our church, my deacon included, took me to doctor's appointments and on errands. I cannot imagine how I would have felt or what my struggle might have been if I did not have God and his willing servants at our church in my life."
>
> Harvey Mednick, Patient, Los Angeles, CA

If You Are an Older Patient

If you are an older person with a chronic medical condition or illness, your faith community will visit you whether you are in a nursing home or at home. Each faith community has groups of people who are in charge of

"It is every Jewish person's responsibility to visit the sick. It is a mitzvah—a holy responsibility to visit the sick. It is not a clergy task alone. We show our support to the patient to let them know 'we are here and we care.'"

Rabbi Morley T. Feinstein,
MAHL, MAHE, DD,
Los Angeles, CA

caring for its members. Volunteers bring food, do marketing, provide trips to the doctor, hospital or pharmacy and visit on a regular basis.

Some nursing homes have a list of ministers, rabbis and other religious professionals whom you can call. These professionals will visit you. All you have to do is ask. This can be a great source of support if you are in need, even if you do not have a preexisting relationship.

If You Are a New Mother

Churches, synagogues and other faith communities also provide help to new mothers. Many will bring food to the new mother's home, arrange for visitors, help with the new baby and more. All you have to do is ask.

If You Need Emotional Support

If a loved one is ill, she may also become depressed and need additional support. You can bring this to your religious professional's attention and request that a phone call or visit be made. Sometimes the comfort of a trusted religious professional is better than anything else for the patient.

Religious institutions also provide emotional support to the family in times of death. Ministers, rabbis and other religious professionals are there to help patients who are ill, but also to help surviving family members.

"One year ago, my cousin went into the hospital for his ninth surgery. He did not survive. He left a wife, four children, a mother and a brother. At that time I was an advocate for the family. I secured a room in the hospital for all of us to talk, worked with the staff so the family could see their loved one, and helped act as a liaison between the family and the hospital bureaucracy. Papers had to be signed, things had to move quickly. I had to be a voice for the voiceless."

Rabbi Morley T. Feinstein, MAHL, MAHE, DD, Los Angeles, CA

Parish Nurses

A parish nurse is a registered nurse who works in a faith community to address health issues for its members and nonmembers alike. She performs health assessments and addresses health needs. She combines the faith of the client with health issues.

A parish nurse can act as a health advisor, health educator, advocate or resource person. As a liaison to faith and community resources, she can answer general health questions. She helps patients create lists of questions to ask their doctors regarding health concerns, upcoming surgeries, procedures and tests. She visits the homebound. A parish nurse offers health education programs and screenings but does not make medical diagnoses or prescribe medications. She helps people to digest and understand medical and health information.

There are also Jewish Congregational Nurses, Muslim Crescent Nurses and many more who serve in similar capacities within other faith traditions.

Medical Advocacy at Religious Institutions

Several religious professionals I spoke with told me about how their congregations connect members who are retired health care providers with members who are in need. There may be a retired nurse or physician in your faith community who can act as your advocate, accompany you to a doctor's appointment, and help you distill medical information. Ask if your religious institution does this. Keep in mind that each religious institution has its own policy about advocacy.

> "Medical advocacy is one of the best things we can do to take care of our members. It is a major part of Christian ministry."
>
> Warren G. Booker Jr, DMin, Lexington, MI

If you have an elderly loved one who is frightened of going to the doctor's office alone, call your religious institution and ask if there is a retired medical professional who might go with her.

According to one minister, this is especially important for vulnerable populations such as the elderly, minorities and the poor.

There are so many good reasons to have an advocate. Beyond the potential for compromised care based on racism or ageism, any patient can

"When someone from church goes with a patient to see a medical professional, it changes the dynamics of the situation with the physician and helps that person gain the confidence to ask questions."

Reverend Warren G. Booker Jr, DMin, Lexington, MI

become nervous in the presence of a medical professional and forget her questions and what she is being told.

Having someone with you also brings more attention to you as the patient and increases the chances of better medical care.

It is a sign of strength to ask for help, whether that be from your religious institution or from a loved one. We all need an advocate at some point in our lives. Speak up!

Referrals

Many churches, synagogues and other faith communities offer referrals to trusted rehabilitation centers, doctors, assisted-living facilities, nursing homes, home health care and more.

How Do I Find Out If My Religious Institution Will Help Me?

"The best thing to do is to reach out to others, whether it is a large or small church. If you're new to the church we might be hesitant to be too pushy. We don't want to overwhelm visitors with what is available. It helps if new people will take the first step to join in."   Jackie Koob, RN, Stanton, CA

If you are a member of a faith community, all you have to do is call or visit your religious professional and ask. If you are not a member of a specific religious institution, call one of interest and ask questions.

PATIENT CHECKLIST

If I am going to have surgery, am in the hospital, recovering at home, in a nursing home, have a chronic medical condition or am a new mother, have I

- ☐ contacted my faith community and religious leader? If I don't have a faith community, do I need to connect with the hospital chaplain?

- ☐ informed my faith community that I need help?

- ☐ asked for someone to accompany me to a doctor's appointment?

- ☐ asked for emotional support?

22

Patient Advocacy

"Some of my patients have caretakers and family members who act as advocates. Having a patient advocate is a definite asset."

ALI TOWFIGH, MD, INTERNAL MEDICINE, WEST LA-VA MEDICAL CENTER, ASSISTANT PROFESSOR OF MEDICINE, UCLA DAVID GEFFEN SCHOOL OF MEDICINE, LOS ANGELES, CA

Enlisting the help of a loved one to act as your advocate is part of getting the best medical care. Even take-charge patients need advocates. An advocate can provide support for you while you see a doctor, be at your bedside if you are in the hospital, help record information offered by a medical professional, converse with you about that information, help you research and more. An advocate is a watchdog as well as someone who gives you confidence because you know that person is at your side and has your best interests at heart.

Advocates act as your eyes and ears to oversee your medical care. If you are in the hospital, have a chronic or serious

"It helps to have a family member or good friend come with the patient. Maybe there is a memory problem, cognitive impairment, or complex medical history. Sometimes patients are deniers or minimizers. It's helpful when a family member or friend comes with the patient to remind the patient of pertinent issues. For example: a patient has sleep apnea. The spouse accompanies the patient and reports symptoms."

Damon Raskin, MD, Internal Medicine, Pacific Palisades, CA

illness, are older or simply need additional support, enlist a family member or good friend to help you. If you have a chronic, serious or perplexing medical situation, bring someone with you to your doctor's appointments. This is to ensure that you get the best medical care.

In choosing an advocate, you'll want to look for someone who is attentive to details, comfortable doing research for and with you and is diplomatic but assertive with medical professionals. You may have several people in mind; think about who would be best at your side during a medical encounter.

What Your Advocate Can Do for You

Ten months into my illness, I started to lose sight of important issues. I was beginning to burn out and felt overwhelmed by the number of doctors I'd seen, by the lack of a correct diagnosis, and fatigued by the chronic pain and by the antibiotics I'd been on for ten months.

I asked a good friend to be my advocate. She is very medically savvy. F. partnered with me as a medical detective. On her own, she researched every diagnosis she could think of. I did the same and then we discussed the viability of each one. We created a plan of action regarding which questions to ask which doctor.

Before I saw each specialist, she and I reviewed my health summary and medical records and created a list of questions for me to ask. She accompanied me to a couple of doctors' appointments. She and I discussed what I had learned from the doctors and which steps to take next. I am very grateful to her.

- Before you see your doctor, ask your advocate to go over any medical records you plan to bring to your visit. Ask her to review your health summary to see if you have included everything. Sometimes when you are in the midst of a medical issue, you can lose sight of the whole picture and forget the details. Stress does that. Also, other people can see things about you or your health that you simply cannot. For example, they see that you have been more fatigued recently or that other behaviors are different.

- Ask your advocate to help you create a list of questions before you see your doctor.

- Ask your advocate to take notes on the conversation with the doctor. Simply ask your physician if it is okay if your advocate takes notes so you can refer to them later. If you are not comfortable having your advocate in the exam room with you, ask her to wait in the waiting room. When you are finished with the doctor, tell her everything the doctor said. Ask her to write it down so you can refer to it later.

- If you have a medical emergency, you can call your advocate and she, in turn, can call your loved ones and alert them to your situation.

- If you are in the hospital, your advocate can show up and help oversee and monitor your care.

- If you need help with language translation, your advocate might be able to assist.

An advocate is your watchdog. Whether you have ongoing medical issues, serious medical issues or you simply need some additional support, enlist a family member or good friend to be your advocate. In turn, you can be an advocate for this person.

> *"My grandmother is not a passive person. As an elderly person who suffers from congestive heart failure, she wants her medical team to talk to her. We as family members are present at doctor visits, and we ask questions, but she makes the decisions. Her health care providers take her seriously because she is active in her care and has us there to support her. We are second in line. We are there to back her up."*
>
> Elizabeth Williams, PhD, Vanderbilt-Ingram Cancer Center, Nashville, TN

How to Create an Advocacy Partnership

If you don't have close family members who live near you, try partnering with another person in your neighborhood and form a mutually beneficial advocacy partnership. This is a two-way street where you serve as advocates for each other. You have her phone number in the case of an emergency and she has yours for the same reason.

Perhaps you are a senior and know another senior who doesn't have a family member living nearby. Suggest creating an advocacy partnership.

You can go to doctors' appointments together and take notes for each other. You can do research for one another. You make a pact. If you are ever in the hospital or in medical need, you know your advocacy partner will be there for you. If there is an emergency, she is the one you will call to oversee and monitor your care. And you will do the same for her.

Put her as an emergency contact on your medical ID card.

How to Find an Advocacy Partner

Here are some ideas on how to find a good match:

- Talk to your physician about this idea. Suggest that she start a list in her office. Maybe one of her staff members can assist in finding other patients who might be interested.

- Your local faith community may be a good place to start. Talk to your faith community leader and ask how you can assist in creating a program like this, where members are matched up with one another as advocacy partners.

- Ask the coordinator at your local senior or community center how you might create an advocacy partners program.

- Neighbors have the advantage of seeing each other on a regular basis. Ask a neighbor with whom you are friendly about the possibility of creating an advocacy partnership.

- Perhaps someone you work with needs an advocate.

- Ask your local hospital how a program like this might be created and how you might be able to help. Start with the patient advocate at the hospital or the head of the volunteer program.

Become an Advocate for Someone in Need

Maybe you have an older or chronically ill neighbor. Perhaps you can check in on this person. Consider asking if she needs something from the market if you are already going. Your neighbor might really be in need but too embarrassed to let you know. Start by offering to lend a hand with a simple task.

Here are a few simple things you can do as an advocate for an older or chronically ill family member, friend or neighbor. These are just suggestions. You must decide what kind of help you can offer based on the time you can spare.

- Offer to pick up something for her at the market when you are going there.

- Offer to take her to the doctor.

- Offer to talk about what she heard from the doctor. Ask her to take notes on her office visit. You can listen and help her distill the information. You can do this after work or after you've gotten the kids to bed.

- Ask her if she would like help creating a list of medications and dosages and what medical conditions she is taking them for. Offer to help organize her medical information.

- Help her create a medical ID card for her wallet. This could be a lifesaver.

If you feel so inclined, you can leave your phone number with her in case of an emergency.

Professional Patient Advocates

Professional patient advocates are specially trained professionals who do research, offer advice, locate medical specialists and generally guide patients and their families through treatment, insurance issues and decision making. Professional patient advocates may also be called nurse navigators or patient navigators. Professional patient advocates can be medical professionals, retired medical professionals or entrepreneurs who are medically savvy and experienced in the medical field. They can help you navigate a complex medical and health care system. They charge a fee.

There are several kinds of professional advocates that patients or caregivers can turn to, including hospital advocates, insurance advocates, case managers, etc. The difference with a private patient advocate is what Trisha

Torrey, author of *Every Patient's Advocate* and founder of AdvoConnection, calls the "allegiance" factor. What she means by this is that whoever pays the advocate will have the advocate's allegiance. If a patient advocate works for you, her allegiance is to you and your needs.

Trisha Torrey also said, "Patients need advocates because the American healthcare system is set up to make money rather than provide care. Not that doctors and hospitals don't want to provide good care—they do—but the pressures put on them by the system that rewards them in many anti-patient ways doesn't allow them to provide premiere care. So if we patients want that excellent care, we need an advocate to help us get it."

PATIENT CHECKLIST

- ☐ Do I need an advocate?

- ☐ If I need an advocate, have I thought about an advocacy partnership?

- ☐ Is there someone I can be an advocate for?

- ☐ Do I want to hire a professional patient advocate?

23

Concierge Doctors
and Patient-Centered Care

*"I couldn't live with the typical way of practicing
medicine any more. I was forced to see too many
patients in too little time. Also, more and more
primary care physicians don't want to see patients in
hospitals; they use hospitalists for that.
In my current practice, I follow patients in the hospital
when they are at their most vulnerable. Frankly, I
couldn't imagine not going to the hospital if one of
my patients was there."*

DAVID BARON, MD, FAMILY MEDICINE, MALIBU, CA,
FORMER CHIEF OF STAFF, SANTA MONICA-UCLA
MEDICAL CENTER & ORTHOPAEDIC HOSPITAL

Concierge Doctors

Concierge doctors will see a certain number of patients for a yearly fee
or retainer. They limit the size of their practices so patients have access to
them when they are in need.

You might be given your concierge doctor's cell phone number and
email address. You will also be given, in most cases, same-day appointments.
Concierge doctors can spend more time with you because they have fewer
patients to see. Many act as advocates and will go with you to see other
doctors.

"I'll do house calls for elderly patients who can't get out of the house."

Damon Raskin, MD,
Internal Medicine,
Pacific Palisades, CA

Most concierge doctors make house calls and many claim that the ability to do so is particularly helpful when it comes to elderly or handicapped patients who have difficulty leaving the house.

Your concierge doctor can coordinate your care with your other doctors. Concierge doctors are actively involved in your care and many claim to be more focused on preventative medical care. They say they are drawn into concierge practices because they want to practice "old-fashioned" medicine.

Other physicians have a concierge component of their practice. They might have a more traditional practice as well as a group of patients who pay for concierge services.

Cost of Concierge Doctors

Fees can range from $1000–$5000 a year and up, depending on the services you want. Many concierge practices have a sliding scale for older patients. You will have to check ahead of time to see whether your insurance plan will pay for their services.

You pay the concierge doctor's yearly fee on top of your health insurance premiums and co-pays.

When asked why he added concierge services to his medical practice, Damon Raskin, MD, said, "I felt that some patients needed more attention. I could give better care to more patients who need it."

Patient-Centered Care

Patient-centered care is based on mutually beneficial partnerships between patients, families and medical providers. This approach to medical care is based on mutual respect and sharing of information with patients and families so they can participate in their medical care. The patient is at the center of the care rather than the physician. Patients and their families are directly involved in decisions involving their treatment.

Patients and their families are encouraged to participate in their care and to collaborate with their medical providers in an effort to improve quality of care and to reduce costs and medical errors. The quality of the relationship between doctor and patient is a cornerstone of patient-centered care, and communication between patients and their medical professionals is crucial to its success. If you use the communication strategies in this book, you'll be well on your way to a patient-centered relationship with your doctor or other medical professional.

Recent studies conclude that if the patient perceives that she is the focus of her medical care then she will recover more quickly and will experience more rapid relief from discomfort or concerns. Improved patient satisfaction and increased patient compliance are also reported results.

Sound familiar? It should, as what I've written about in this book shares some similarities to patient-centered care.

What can hinder patient-centered care is the time constraint between most doctors and their patients in office visits. It takes time to develop a relationship, and if a doctor takes health insurance, she is forced to see many patients in a day simply to cover her costs. This minimizes the time each doctor can spend with patients.

Accountable Care Organizations

Accountable care organizations (ACOs) are based on the concept of patient-centered care. An ACO is a group of medical providers such as hospitals, long-term care facilities, physicians and other medical professionals that all work together to coordinate care for their Medicare patients who have the original Medicare plan. The focus of ACOs is on patients and their providers partnering on care decisions. One goal of ACOs is to improve quality of care and reduce fragmented medical care for those with more than one doctor. ACOs are patient-centered organizations.

Patient-Centered Medical Home

Patient-centered medical home is an approach to patient care in which a team of medical professionals provides patients with coordinated care throughout their lifetime. Each patient has a personal physician who leads a coordinated and integrated team that views the patient as a whole. Services include prevention, treatment of acute and chronic illness, and assistance with end-of-life issues.

Patients enrolled in a medical home program are expected to develop long-term relationships with their primary care physicians who coordinate their care with specialists and ensure that they get the appointments they need.

Quality and safety are hallmarks of the patient-centered medical home.

The patient is the focus of the health care delivery system and the aim is to remove the wall between medical professionals and patients. The physician is accessible to the patient and often gets to know patients' families and lifestyle.

PATIENT CHECKLIST

- ☐ Do I want a concierge doctor?

- ☐ If I want a concierge doctor, have I found referrals?

- ☐ Have I researched the credentials of the concierge doctor I am considering?

- ☐ Have I called the concierge doctor's office and asked if she takes my insurance?

- ☐ Have I inquired about the concierge doctor's fees?

- ☐ Have I asked if a doctor I already see has a concierge component to her practice?

- ☐ Do I want a patient-centered physician?

- ☐ Do I want patient-centered care?

- ☐ Do I want a patient-centered medical home?

24

Telemedicine and Telehealth
The wave of the future

"Wireless health may be defined as the use of wireless technologies for education, health management, and public safety. It encompasses solutions that facilitate continuous access to health care information, expert advice, or therapeutic intervention enabled by telecommunication networks. Telehealth is but one example. This industry will become an integral and essential part of fitness and healthcare in the near future, spawned by the perfect storm of prohibitive healthcare costs, a shortage of physicians, and remarkable developments in nanotechnology, biological sensors, and genomic medicine."

DAVID LEE SCHER, MD, FACC, FHRS, HARRISBURG, PA

Telemedicine

A growing trend, telemedicine is the use of medical information sent from one site to another via electronic communications to improve patients' health status. Telemedicine refers to remote delivery of health care. For example, you or your doctor can have a consultation with a specialist across the world. Medical records and images are sent for diagnoses and treatment plans. Email, video conferencing, wireless phones and more are used for the transmission.

"Telemedicine can be as simple as two health professionals discussing a case over the telephone, or as complex as using internet technologies to conduct a real-time, face-to-face consultation between patient and doctor or between medical specialists in two different countries. Telemedicine generally refers to the use of communications and information technologies, particularly the internet, for the transmission and interchange of personal health data for storage and for clinical care."

Louis Siegel, MD,
Lakewood Ranch, FL

This means that you can have a consultation with a specialist who is the best match to diagnose and treat your medical condition, regardless of your location. In addition, you and your doctor can communicate with this specialist who is located far from your city and transmit your diagnostic images and/or video along with your medical records in order to get her opinion. This may involve having a consult with a physician via a live video transmission like Skype™.

This is fantastic news for patients who cannot travel or for those living in the rural areas without access to good care. It's even beneficial for those in metropolitan areas who simply need an expert who lives across the country.

There's even more to it.

Telemedicine is practicing medicine at a distance, enabled by technology and high-speed telecommunication networks. It can improve patient compliance and continuity of care. Telemedicine is about expanding access to information.

Telemedicine can also connect geographically separated health care organizations to improve education and medical care.

In a nutshell, telemedicine can offer

- access for physicians to consult remotely;
- tele-imaging of patient records and files;
- remote clinical diagnostics;
- support for surgical procedures.

The Advantages of Telemedicine

Telemedicine increases access to health care. Remote patients can more easily obtain clinical services. Home monitoring can reduce the cost of hospital stays. Rural physicians can have access to specialists and to more education.

If you live in a rural area and don't have access to medical school-affiliated doctors and specialists, telemedicine might be helpful to you. It can also benefit patients who have an illness or injury that prevents them from traveling.

If you have a wound and are unable to see your doctor for an office visit, or you are traveling, consider asking your doctor if you can send a digital photo or video of your wound to her. She might be able to advise you on the problem.

Computers and smartphones are equipped with cameras, speakers and microphones, allowing providers and patients to see and hear each other even when separated by large distances. Some computers and smartphones have attachments that allow doctors to remotely look into a patient's ear, perform an ultrasound, listen to a patient's lungs and heart, and much more.

By using robotic devices, a surgeon can even assist with surgery that is performed in a different country.

A Potential Downside of Telemedicine

Several doctors said that telemedicine minimizes and restricts the doctor-patient encounter. Many doctors emphasized the need to see the patient in person. Telemedicine puts distance between patients and their doctors and could adversely affect the doctor-patient relationship.

Telehealth

Telehealth is an expansion on telemedicine. It includes the support of long-distance clinical health care, patient and professional health-related education, public health and health administration. Videoconferencing, the internet, streaming and wireless communications are used.

Remote patient monitoring is included under the umbrella of telehealth and focuses on devices that are used to collect data to monitor a patient's status. For example, a patient may

"One possible disadvantage is that some of the 'human elements' of delivering healthcare may be missing when care is delivered remotely. Can a doctor completely sense your level of worry and fear merely by seeing your face on a computer screen? Can you, as a patient, receive the comfort and reassurance you need when the doctor is unable to hold your hand or put her arm around you?"

Louis Siegel, MD,
Lakewood Ranch, FL

have a pacemaker that is equipped to send signals to her doctor or to a monitoring service that keeps track of her heart rhythms. The monitoring service can be interactive.

mHealth

mHealth, or mobile health, is the practice of medicine supported by devices such as mobile phones and PDAs. mHealth employs communication technology in the exchange of information via a mobile device.

The beauty of mHealth is that devices such as mobile phones are potentially accessible to almost everyone regardless of financial or social status because most everyone can carry a mobile phone.

mHealth has emerged in recent years largely as an application for developing countries, stemming from the rapid rise of mobile phone penetration in low-income nations. Information can reach lower-income and rural areas, populations that generally receive less than optimum medical care.

mHealth offers increased access to health care and health-related information for hard-to-reach populations. It allows for improved ability to diagnose and track diseases. It can provide current public health information to remote locations and expanded access to ongoing medical education.

mHealth has great potential to promote better health communication to encourage healthier lifestyles and to increase patient compliance, diagnostic and treatment support, remote monitoring, remote data collection and much more.

Amazing, isn't it?

eHealth

eHealth is a relatively new term that seems to lack an agreed-upon definition. According to the World Health Organization, eHealth is the use of electronic information technology in the health sector.

e-Patient

e-patient is a term coined in the 1990s to describe patients who used the newly available internet to bring new value to their health care situation by finding information and other patients and families with whom they could share information.

Tom Ferguson originally defined e-patients as empowered, equipped and engaged in their health care decisions. Ferguson died in 2006, and in 2009 his friends and followers incorporated the Society for Participatory Medicine.

Dave deBronkart, known as "e-Patient Dave," is the leading spokesperson for the e-patient movement. A high-tech executive and online community leader for many years, he was diagnosed in 2007 with Stage IV kidney cancer, with median survival of twenty-four weeks. He used the internet in every way possible to partner with his care team. Today he is well. Dave deBronkart learned to use every aspect of empowerment, technology and participatory medicine to fight his disease.

PATIENT CHECKLIST

☐ Do I need a second opinion via teleconferencing from a specialist who does not live in my city?

☐ If I want a second opinion with a specialist who doesn't live in my city, have I gotten referrals for specialists who are the best to treat my condition, illness or disease?

☐ Did I do research on the doctors I was referred to?

☐ Did I call the doctors' offices and ask if they do consults via telephone, Skype™ or some other method of videoconferencing?

☐ Have I asked about fees for this type of consultation?

☐ If I have an appointment for remote medical care with a specialist, have I discussed it with my primary care physician?

☐ Have I sent the specialist copies of my pertinent medical records?

☐ Have I called the specialist's office to make sure my medical records arrived?

25

Why It Is Essential to Create
Your Legal Health Documents Now

*"The time to have end-of-life discussions is when you
are in mint condition."*

JESSICA G. SCHAIRER, PHD, CLINICAL AND HEALTH PSYCHOLOGIST,
LOS ANGELES, CA

We must prepare now in case we are ever seriously ill, injured or cannot speak for ourselves. These are uncomfortable issues to talk about and most of us don't even like to think about them. But I believe that preparation of documents such as advance directive, living will and durable power of attorney for health care is the ultimate act of advocacy for oneself. As take-charge patients, we make the time to execute these documents.

> "The prepared patient thinks about end-of-life issues early on. It eases family members' minds about what to do."
>
> Jack C. Rosenfeld, MD,
> Family Medicine and
> Geriatrics, Lansdale, PA

These legal documents ensure that you will receive the kind of medical care you want if you become very ill or seriously injured. If you create these documents with the help of an attorney or legal organization, you will be in the driver's seat regarding what happens to you if you are incapable of directing your medical care.

Create Your Legal Health Documents Now

The time to prepare these documents is when you are healthy, not when you are sick or injured. It is never easy to address these issues.

Advance Directive

With the help of an attorney or legal organization, create this document to state your choice for what kind of medical treatment and intervention you want in the face of serious illness or serious injury. You can also appoint someone to make that choice if you are unable to do it for yourself. This avoids confusion

> "People have to be more proactive about end-of-life choices."
>
> Lauren Fite, Physician's Assistant, Los Angeles, CA

later on and ensures that you get the kind of medical care and treatment you think is right for you.

Living Will

This is a document in which you state the kind of life-prolonging medical care you want if you become terminally ill, permanently unconscious or are unable to make your own decisions.

Durable Power of Attorney for Health Care

This is another kind of advance directive. It names a person to make medical decisions for you if you are unable to.

Do Not Resuscitate (DNR)

This is a document that states that you do not want resuscitation (CPR) if your heart stops beating or you stop breathing. Give a copy to your PCP.

My mother and godmother were in the hospital for extended stays and I know in my heart that neither of them would have wanted what happened to them if they had known ahead of time. Everything was done medically to prolong their lives, which in the end prolonged their suffering. My mother was in the hospital for five months, on full life support for several of those months, and my godmother was in the hospital for seven months, also on full life support for a few of those months. Now, these are extreme situations, but if you have ever witnessed a loved one's suffering and were unable to do anything about it, you know that you would never want that for yourself.

Right after my mother passed away, I marched myself down to my attorney's office to create all the necessary documents. I was determined never to allow myself to be in the same position my mother was, and I certainly did not want my family struggling with stressful decisions regarding my medical care. If I am sick or injured, they are going to be stressed enough.

Discuss Your Wishes with Your Doctor and Loved Ones

Talk to your primary care physician. Discussing your wishes with her is extremely important. Give her copies of these legal documents so she will know what to do for you.

Talk to a trusted loved one. Discuss your wishes with your spouse, partner or a close family member. Explain to them what you want for yourself in the event of a medical emergency, serious illness or injury.

> "It's one of the more important things I do–letting people die with dignity. It's one of the hardest things I do. You feel the patient's and the family's pain. I care about them."
>
> Jo Ann C. Pullen, MD, Internal Medicine and Geriatrics, Los Angeles, CA

You may not feel comfortable talking to anyone about these issues. This is very understandable. However, this is about being a take-charge patient and end-of-life issues are a part of your health care. You may not want life-prolonging measures or you might want everything possible to be done to keep you alive. How is anyone going to know this unless you tell them?

Learn about Palliative Care and Hospice Care

Several doctors said that it is difficult for them to discuss end-of-life issues with their patients. As difficult as these topics are to think about, you might want to initiate a conversation with your doctor about how you want to be treated at the end of your life.

Palliative Care

The goal of palliative care is to relieve suffering and improve quality of life for people of all ages with serious, chronic and life-threatening illnesses. It is not the same as hospice. It involves a team of doctors, nurses, social workers, psychologists, dieticians and religious professionals who support the patient.

It is not about giving up hope for recovery. Some patients recover and move out of palliative care.

Hospice Care

Hospice provides support for people entering the final stages of their lives. It strives to enhance the quality of a person's life by providing medical care, pain management and psychological or spiritual support. Hospice care is comfort care only. It is intended for patients with terminal illnesses who have exhausted all curative and therapeutic treatments.

Most hospice care takes place in the home, but it can also be delivered in a nursing home or hospice care facility. Some evidence suggests that hospice care can actually extend life.

Topics to Discuss with Your Doctor

- Ask your doctor to explain palliative care and hospice care to you.
- Explain to your doctor what quality of life means to you. This includes how you feel about aggressive medical treatments, life support, quality time with your loved ones and where you want to have your treatments.
- Explain any of your religious or spiritual beliefs and cultural values that are important to your care.

Inform your doctor if you have executed an advance directive, a living will, durable power of attorney for health care or DNR. If you have, provide her with a copy or each.

PATIENT CHECKLIST

- ☐ Did I create my advance directive, living will and durable power of attorney for health care?

- ☐ Have I given copies of these legal documents to my primary care physician?

- ☐ Have I discussed my wishes with my primary care doctor and a trusted love one?

Definitions

Medical Professionals

Doctor of Medicine (MD): A physician who has had many years of training including four years of undergraduate education, four years of medical school, and who received an MD degree after passing exams. The requirements for an MD degree vary in other countries.

Primary Care Physician (PCP): A medical doctor who provides continuing care of a variety of medical conditions. Primary care physicians provide diagnosis and treatment of common illnesses and medical conditions. They are usually the first point of care for patients. The PCP takes your history, does physical examinations, annual checkups, screenings, immunizations, orders tests and interprets the results, diagnoses and treats illnesses and injuries; educates patients about preventative medicine and healthy living.

Specialist: A doctor who has had advanced education and full-time training in an accredited residency program for her specific medical field. If you have an HMO, you must be referred to an in-network specialist by your PCP.

Board-Certified Doctor: A doctor who has completed an approved educational program and an advanced training program and has passed rigid examinations required by a medical specialty board. Once the doctor completes these certification requirements, she becomes board certified. Doctors who complete all certification requirements except the examination are called "board eligible."

Surgeon: The doctor who operates on a patient who is having surgery.

Hospitalist: A hospital doctor who cares for all hospitalized patients.

Intensivist: A hospital doctor assigned to take care of all critical care patients in the hospital.

Doctor of Osteopathy (DO): A medical doctor who holds a DO degree and is known as an osteopathic physician. The DO has similar education and training as an MD but receives training in the body's musculoskeletal system and osteopathic manipulative treatment.

Physician's Assistant (PA): A health care professional who is licensed to practice medicine under the supervision of a licensed physician. The PA has a similar role to a physician and performs physical exams, diagnoses and treats illness and injury, orders and interprets tests, encourages preventative health care, and can write prescriptions in some states. Most physician's assistant programs require both two years of college in an accredited program and advanced health care training. The Physician Assistant National Certification Exam must be passed to obtain a license. The requirements for a PA vary from state to state.

Nurse Practitioner (NP): A registered nurse who has completed advanced nursing education (usually a master's degree) and extensive clinical training in the diagnosis, management, treatment and prevention of medical conditions. An NP provides complete physical examinations, diagnoses and treats medical conditions, orders tests, prescribes and manages patient medication and emphasizes preventative care and health maintenance. States have different requirements for NPs.

Registered Nurse (RN): A health care professional who graduated from a state-approved nursing program and passed the National Council Licensure Examination for Registered Nurses. Training to become an RN includes both academic and hands-on experience. An RN might work in a hospital, outpatient urgent care center, doctor's office, operating room, or intensive care unit. An RN oversees work of other caregivers such as LPNs and LVNs.

Licensed Practical Nurse (LPN) or Licensed Vocational Nurse (LVN): A nursing professional who usually works under the supervision of an

RN. An LPN is required to take a one- to two-year vocational training program and pass the NCLEX-PN practical nurse test to become certified. An LPN provides varied and valuable services in hospitals, skilled nursing homes, medical offices, and home health care.

Tests and Scans

Angiography or Arteriography: A procedure used to reveal the inside of organs and blood vessels in the body. It shows the arteries in many areas in the body as well as veins and heart chambers. This diagnostic test can identify blood clots, blockages, and tumors.

Biopsy: A procedure to remove and examine a tissue sample from a living body for diagnostic purposes. Many biopsies are done to determine whether or not a patient has a cancer.

Colonoscopy: A procedure used to examine the entire colon. An instrument called a colonoscope is used which can view the lining of the colon and the rectum. This test helps diagnose colon cancer, polyps, unexplained abdominal pain and symptoms, bowel disease and tumors.

CT Scan: Computerized tomography scan. This scan takes cross-sectional images of structures and soft tissue in the body that cannot be seen in conventional x-rays. This scan can show disease or abnormalities in tissue and bone.

Echocardiogram: A test that uses sound waves to create a moving picture of the heart. The picture is much more detailed than a plain x-ray image and involves no radiation exposure.

Mammography: An x-ray that examines breast tissue and which is used as both a screening and diagnostic tool. It is used to detect breast masses, calcifications and cancer.

MRI: Magnetic resonance imaging. An MRI uses a magnetic field and radio waves to take detailed 3-D images of the tissues and organs in the body. It is used to find both benign and malignant tumors, abnormal tissue, changes or bleeding in the brain and other problems.

PET Scan: Positron emission tomography scan. This scan distinguishes between normal cells and cancer cells. PET scans are often used for follow-up to see if a tumor is cancerous or not.

Ultrasound: A technique using high-frequency sound waves. An ultrasound allows physicians get an inside view of soft tissues and body cavities. It is also referred to as a sonogram.

Upper Endoscopy: A procedure used to examine the inside of the body. A lighted, flexible instrument known as an endoscope is introduced through the mouth. It examines the esophagus, stomach, and duodenum. This test can help diagnose the cause of gastrointestinal bleeding, stomach pain, ulcers, and tumors.

Resources

Here is a list of resources to help you. For an updated list of resources, please visit the Resources section at www.thetakechargepatient.com.

General Health Information

- American Academy of Family Practice
  http://www.aafp.org/
- American Academy of Pediatrics
  http://www.aap.org/
- American College of Physicians
  http://www.acponline.org/
- American Medical Association
  http://www.ama-assn.org/
- American Red Cross
  http://www.redcross.org
- Consumer Reports (subscription required)
  http://consumerreports.org/health/home.htm
- Family Doctor
  http://familydoctor.org/online/famdocen/home.html
- Johns Hopkins Health Alerts
  http://www.johnshopkinshealthalerts.com/
- Livestrong: Lance Armstrong's Foundation
  http://www.livestrong.com/

- The Merck Manuals Online Medical Library
  http://merckmanuals.com/professional/index.html
- Merck Medicus
  http://www.merckmedicus.com/pp/us/hcp/hcp_home.jsp
- University of California at Berkeley wellness site
  http://www.wellnessletter.com/
- Up To Date
  http://www.uptodate.com/patients/index.html

Medical Schools

- Harvard Medical School
  http://hms.harvard.edu/hms/home.asp
- Stanford School of Medicine
  http://med.stanford.edu/
- UCLA Medical Center
  http://www.ucla.edu/
- University of California at Los Angeles health site
  http://www.uclahealth.org/
  http://www.ucla.edu/research.html/

Clinics and Hospitals

- Cleveland Clinic Website
  http://my.clevelandclinic.org/default.aspx
- The Mayo Clinic
  http://www.mayoclinic.com/
- MD Anderson Cancer Center in Houston, Texas
  http://www.mdanderson.org/
- Memorial Sloan-Kettering Cancer Center
  http://www.mskcc.org/mskcc/html/44.cfm
- Scripps in San Diego, California
  http://www.scripps.org/

Government Health Resources

- AHRQ, Agency for Healthcare Research and Quality
  http://www.ahrq.gov/
- Centers for Disease Control and Prevention
  http://www.cdc.gov/
- Health.gov
  http://health.gov/
- Health Finder.gov
  http://www.healthfinder.gov/
- HHS.Gov
  http://www.hhs.gov/
- Medline Plus
  http://www.nlm.nih.giv/medlineplus/
- National Institutes of Health
  http://nih.gov/
- U.S. Food and Drug Administration
  http://fda.gov/
- U.S. National Library of Medicine & National Institutes of Health
  Pub Med
  http://www.ncbi.nlm.nih.gov/pubmed/
- World Health Organization (WHO)
  http://www.who.int/en/

Diseases and Conditions

- American Cancer Society
  http://www.cancer.org/
- American Diabetes Association
  http://www.diabetes.org/
- American Heart Association
  http://www.heart.org/

- American Lung Association
  http://www.lungusa.org/
- City of Hope
  http://www.cityofhope.org
- Clinical Trials
  http://clinicaltrials.gov/
- Cure Together
  http://www.curetogether.com/
- National Cancer Institute
  http://www.cancer.gov/
- National Institutes of Health—Office of Rare Diseases Research
  http://rarediseases.info.nih.gov/

Senior Resources

- American Association of Retired Persons
  http://www.aarp.org/
- Assisted Living Federation of America
  http://www.alfa.org
- Caring For Your Parents
  http://www.pbs.org/wgbh/caringforyourparents/
- Center For Healthy Aging
  http://www.healthyagingprograms.org/
- Leading Age
  http://aahsa.org/
- Medicare
  www.medicare.gov/
- ParentGiving
  http://www.parentgiving.com/

Drug Safety

- Consumer Reports (subscription required)
  http://www.consumerreports.org/health/prescription_drugs/index
  .htm
- Drugs.Com
  http://www.drugs.com/
- Epocrates
  http://www.epocrates.com/
- Safe Medication
  http://www.safemedication.com/
- U.S. Food and Drug Administration
  http://www.fda.gov

Hospitals

- American Hospital Association
  http://www.aha.gov/
- Consumer Reports Hospital Ratings (subscription required)
  http://www.consumerreports.org/health/doctors-hospitals/
  doctorsand-hospitals.htm
- HealthGrades
  http://www.healthgrades.com/
- Hospital Compare
  U.S. Department of Health and Human Services
  http://www.hospitalcompare.hhs.gov/
- The Joint Commission
  http://www.jointcommission.org/
- The LeapFrog Group
  http://www.leapfroggroup.org/cp

Recommended Books

The Eldercare Handbook by Stella Morea Henry

The Empowered Patient: Hundreds of Life-Saving Facts, Action Steps and Strategies You Need to Know by Dr. Julia Hallisy

The Empowered Patient: How to Get the Right Diagnosis, Buy the Cheapest Drugs, Beat Your Insurance Company, and Get the Best Medical Care Every Time by Elizabeth Cohen

How Doctors Think by Jerome Groopman, MD

Laugh, Sing, and Eat Like a Pig: How an Empowered Patient Beat Stage IV Cancer by Dave deBronkart

The Mayo Clinic Family Health Book

Routine Miracles by Conrad Fischer, MD

The Savvy Patient by Mark Pettus

You Bet Your Life! The 10 Mistakes Every Patient Makes by Trisha Torrey

You: The Smart Patient by Michael F. Roizen, MD, and Mehmet C. Oz, MD

References

Books

Bernay, Toni, Ph.D, and Saar Porrath, M.D. (2006). *When It's Cancer: The 10 Essential Steps to Follow after Your Diagnosis.* New York: Holtzbrinck Publishers.

Fischer, Conrad M.D. (2009). *Routine Miracles: Personal Journeys of Patients and Doctors Discovering the Powers of Modern Medicine.* New York: Kaplan Publishing.

Groopman, Jerome E. (2008). *How Doctors Think.* New York: Houghton Mifflin.

Roizen, Michael F. M.D., and Mehmet C. Oz, M.D. (2006). *You: The Smart Patient: An Insider's Guide for Getting the Best Treatment.* New York: Free Press.

Sanders, Lisa, M.D. (2009). *Every Patient Tells a Story: Medical Mysteries and the Art of Diagnosis.* New York: Broadway Books.

Articles

Abelson, Reed (2010, September 7). Another kind of medical error. *The New York Times.* Retrieved December 5, 2011 from http://prescriptions.blogs.nytimes.com/2010/09/07/another-kind-of-medical-error/

Bakalar, Nicholas (2009, June 22). Abnormal test results may not get to patients. *The New York Times.* Retrieved December 5, 2011 from http://www.nytimes.com/2009/06/23/health/23patient.html

Baldauf, Sarah (2010, April 30). Patient advocate: Bring a friend to the hospital. *U.S. News & World Report*. Retrieved December 5, 2011 from http://health.usnews.com/health-news/managing-your-healthcare/healthcare/articles/2010/04/30/patient-advocate-bring-a-friend-to-the-hospital

Bonvissuto, Kimberly (2010, June 4). Expanding medicine beyond physicians' office walls. Retrieved December 5, 2011 from http://www.modernmedicine.com/modernmedicine/article/articleDetail.jsp?id=673929

Brody, Nicholas (n.d.). The rise of the empowered patient. *Scientific American Pathways*. Retrieved November 18, 2011 from http://www.sa-pathways.com/new-health-consumer/the-rise-of-the-empowered-patient

Cantlupe, Joe (2011, May 26). Patient safety needs a rescue. Retrieved November 18, 2011 from http://www.healthleadersmedia.com/page-1/PHY-266648/Patient-Safety-Needs-a-Rescue

Clancy, Carolyn M., M.D. (2008, February 5). Navigating the health care system. Retrieved November 18, 2011 from http://www.ahrq.gov/consumer/cc/cc020508.htm

Crane, Mark (2010, June 28). New study finds 91% of physicians practice defensive medicine. Medscape Medical News. Retrieved November 18, 2011 from http://www.medscape.com/viewarticle/724254

Dead by mistake (n.d.). timesunion.com. Retrieved December 6, 2011 from http://www.timesunion.com/deadbymistake/

'Difficult' patients more likely to experience worse symptoms (2011, January 26). Retrieved November 18, 2011 from http://www.sciencedaily.com/releases/2011/01/110126081603.htm

Dolan, Pamela Lewis (2010, January 18). Participatory medicine: A high-tech alliance with patients. Retrieved December 5, 2011 from http://www.amaassn.org/amednews/2010/01/18/bisa0118.htm

Elejalde-Ruiz, Alexia (2010, June 24). It'll only hurt for a minute. *Chicago Tribune*. Retrieved November 18, 2011 from http://articles.chicagotribune.com/2010-06-24/health/sc-cons-0624-

save-negotiate-medical-c20100624_1_medical-bills-medical-care-doctor

Finding Dr. Right (2011, March). *Consumer Reports*. Retrieved November 18, 2011 from http://www.consumerreports.org/cro/magazine-archive/2011/march/health/doctors/finding-dr-right/index.htm

Gallagher, Thomas H., M.D., Amy D. Waterman, Ph.D, Alison G. Ebers, and Victoria J. Fraser, M.D. (2003). Patients' and physicians' attitudes regarding the disclosure of medical errors [Electronic version]. *Journal of the American Medical Association*, 289(8), 1001-1007.

Getlen, Larry (n.d.). Fighting health insurance claim denials. Retrieved November 18, 2011 from http://www.bankrate.com/finance/insurance/fighting-health-insurance-claim-denials-1.aspx

HealthGrades seventh annual patient safety in American hospitals study (2010, March). Retrieved November 21, 2011 from http://www.healthgrades.com/media/DMS/pdf/PatientSafetyInAmericanHospitalsStudy2010.pdf

Health insurer preauthorization policies affecting patient care. (2010, December 8). AMAWlre. Retrieved November 18, 2011 from http://www.ama-assn.org/ama/pub/amawire/2010-december-08.shtml

How to cut wait time at the doctor's office (2010, October 20). CBS News. Retrieved December 5, 2011 from http://www.cbsnews.com/stories/2010/10/20/earlyshow/health/main6975069.shtml

Huntington, Beth BSN, MSN, JD, and Nettie Kuhn, RN, BSPA, CPHRM (2003). Communication gaffes: A root cause of malpractice claims [Electronic version]. *Baylor University Medical Center Proceedings*, 16(2), 157-161.

IT helps to prevent misdiagnosis (2007, August 31). Retrieved December 5, 2011 from http://www.medicalnewstoday.com/releases/80903.php

Landro, Laura (2011, August 16). When a doctor isn't enough. *The Wall Street Journal*. Retrieved November 18, 2011 from http://

online.wsj.com/article/SB1000142405311190425320457651104728
28240848.html

Landro, Laura (2011, December 6). Bigger roles for chaplains
on patient medical teams. *The Wall Street Journal.* Retrieved
December 7, 2011 from http://online.wsj.com/article/SB10001424
052970204826704577074462494881428.html?mod=googlenews_
wsj

Levinson, Wendy, M.D., Debra L. Roter, Ph.D, John P. Mullooly,
Ph.D, Valerie T. Dull, Ph.D, and Richard M. Frankel, Ph.D
(1997). The relationship with malpractice claims among
primary care physicians and surgeons. *The Journal of the
American Medical Association,* 277(7), 553-559. Abstract
retrieved December 5, 2011 from http://jama.ama-assn.org/
content/277/7/553.abstract

Lickerman, Alex,   (n.d.). Help doctors to best care for their patients.
Retrieved November 18, 2011 from http://www.kevinmd.com/
blog/2010/03/doctors-care-patients.html

Look-and-sound-alike names account for many painkiller
prescription errors (2011, February 1). *U.S. News & World
Report.* Retrieved December 5, 2011 from http://health.usnews.
com/health-news/family-health/pain/articles/2011/02/01/
look-and-sound-alike-names-account-for-many-painkiller-
prescription-errors

Lowes, Robert (2009, June 4). Retainer physicians help uninsured
but face legal obstacles. Medscape Medical News. Retrieved
November 18, 2011 from http://www.medscape.com/
viewarticle/703900

Medication errors injure 1.5 million people and cost billions of
dollars annually (2006, July 20). Retrieved December 6, 2011
from http://www8.nationalacademies.org/onpinews/newsitem.
aspx?recordid=11623

Miller, Henry (2011, February 16). Medication mistakes are a tough
pill to swallow. *Forbes.* Retrieved December 5, 2011 from http://
www.forbes.com/sites/henrymiller/2011/02/16/medication-
mistakes-are-a-tough-pill-to-swallow/

Parker-Pope, Tara (2008, July 29). Doctor and patient, now at
  odds. *The New York Times*. Retrieved December 6, 2011from
  http://www.nytimes.com/2008/07/29/health/29well.html?_
  r=4&adxnnl=1&oref=slogin&adxnnlx=1217426510-jC7WeEHM
  15TC4T3LLSSf2A&oref=slogin&oref=slogin
Patient centered medical home can change the way care is delivered
  (2009, June 1). Retrieved November 18, 2011 from http://www.
  ehealthnews.eu/ibm/1621-patient-centered-medical-home-can-
  change-the-way-care-is-delivered
Receiving patient centered care: Top ten things a patient or
  family member can do to ensure quality care (n.d.) PBS.
  org. Retrieved December 5, 2011 from http://www.pbs.org/
  remakingamericanmedicine/ensure.html
Torrey, Trisha (2011, April 11). How to correct errors in your
  medical records: These mistakes can affect your healthcare
  and outcomes. Retrieved November 18, 2011 from http://
  patients.about.com/od/yourmedicalrecords/a/howtocorrect.htm
Tribble, Sarah Jane (2009, June 02). The health-care industry's new
  hope: Patient-centered care. Cleveland.com. Retrieved November
  18, 2011 from http://www.cleveland.com/healthfit/index.
  ssf/2009/06/_str_proposed_headline_the.html
Weed, Julie (2009, June 6). If all doctors had more time to listen. *The
  New York Times*. Retrieved December 5, 2011 from http://www.
  nytimes.com/2009/06/07/health/07health.html?pagewanted=all
Weinick, Robin M., Rachel M. Burns and Ateev Mehrotra (2010,
  September). Many emergency department visits could be
  managed at urgent care centers and retail clinics. *Health Affairs*,
  29(9), 1630-1636. Abstract retrieved December 5, 2011 from
  http://content.healthaffairs.org/content/29/9/1630.abstract
What doctors wish their patients knew (2011, February 8). Consumer
  Reports.org. Retrieved November 18, 2011 from http://
  pressroom.consumerreports.org/pressroom/2011/02/plus-how-
  technology-can-transform-primary-care-yonkers-ny-doctors-
  reveal-what-patients-can-do-to-get-better-care-in-a.html

WhiteCoat, MD (2010, September). Mail order pharmacies have cheap prices, but also problems. Retrieved December 5, 2011 from http://www.kevinmd.com/blog/2010/09/mail-order-pharmacies-cheap-prices-problems.html

Acknowledgments

A book is never written alone, and I had wonderful help with this one. Many physicians, other medical professionals, patients and patients' loved ones were very generous with their time, knowledge and resources. They offered not only very interesting and credible information but also fascinating personal stories. Each provided a unique perspective on health care, and few expected much in return for their contributions. I thank each one and express my deepest gratitude, because without them, this book never would have been written.

The following physicians and other professionals contributed far more than their share and willingly went the extra mile to help *The Take-Charge Patient* become the best it could be. Many thanks to Jack C. Rosenfeld MD, Jo Ann C. Pullen MD, Zouhdi A. Hajjaj MD, Fran Ginsberg, Lawrence S. Miller MD, David A. Rapkin PhD, Cheri Adrian PhD, Roger E. Dafter PhD, Elizabeth A. Williams PhD, H. Kenneth Schueler, Peter Naysan PharmD, Arian Moini PharmD, Joseph J. Morgan MD, Robert J. Adair MD, Sheryl A. Ross MD, Daniel Wohlgelernter MD, Jackie Koob RN, David Lee Scher MD, Damon Raskin MD, David Baron MD, Peter Angood MD and Bernard P. Ginsberg MD.

To all of the fearless patients who contributed to this book—thank you for sharing your personal stories.

I spent a rough sixteen months trying to find a diagnosis and cure for a chronic pain condition. I am very grateful to my family and good friends for supporting me throughout the process. Heartfelt thanks go to my husband,

Jamie—you loved, supported and cared for me every step of the way—you are simply the best. To Fran Ginsberg, you are an amazing advocate, good friend and medical researcher extraordinaire. Words cannot do justice to my appreciation for all of your support and hard work. To Lucy, I am very lucky to have a daughter who is so sweet and was so supportive during such a trying time. To my stepson, Logan, your empathy and support meant a lot to me. To my dear friend Rachel Ballon, you were there to listen, talk, laugh and cry with me all those months; your support meant more to me than words can say. To my dear and cherished friend Loren Alison, your support, compassion and insights spurred me on.

Many, many thanks to Sarah Gallwey, Lisa Deeb, Melissa Browne, Marge Ehrenclou, Gail Uellendahl, Annika Baker, Judy Chambers Beck, Sally Marshi, Randi Kinsler, Victoria Bloch, Winnie Wechsler, Debbie Berman, Linda Newton, Barbara Cadow, Annie Behringer, Lauree Berger Turman, Janet Pucino, Marlu Harris, Harvey Mednick, Jessie Browne, Nancy Stark, Mimi Daly, and Sarah Lewis.

A special note of gratitude to Dr. Shirin Towfigh for not only diagnosing me correctly and curing me of my pain but also for your wonderful care—and for performing surgery on a Saturday morning when you didn't have to.

A sincere expression of thanks to Dr. Amy Rosenman, who provided such good, collaborative care, tending to my medical needs on short notice—you certainly went all out for me on a number of occasions. You and your staff are the best.

Much appreciation to Dr. William Pullen, who practices such good patient-centered care. Thank you for not losing your sense of humor when I certainly had lost mine.

A very special thanks to Alan Gadney for guiding and helping me get this book to print and beyond. A big thank you to Benita Gold and to those people who took a special interest in promoting this book—you know who you are.

Finally, to the very important and talented professionals who designed, edited and indexed this book—my deepest thanks for doing a fantastic job—George Foster, Kristin Langenfeld, Sue Knopf and Rachel Rice.

Patient Safety Checklists
and
Sample Questions
for Yourself and Your Doctor

The following patient safety checklists are provided for your use.
Please feel free to photocopy them.

Medication Safety Checklist for Patients

☐ Do I know the name and dosage of the medication my doctor prescribed?

☐ Do I understand why I am taking this medication?

☐ Do I understand how to take this medication?

☐ Do I know the brand and generic names of this medication?

☐ Did I review the prescription in the doctor's office?

☐ Did I look at the medication at the pharmacy?

☐ Do I need to set up an appointment to meet with my pharmacist?

☐ Do I need help managing my medications?

☐ Have I explored my options to get help to manage my medications?

☐ Have I created a list of all my medications?

☐ Have I considered using only one pharmacy?

☐ Do I need to set up timers to alert me to take my medications?

☐ Have I provided a list of my medication allergies to my physicians, other medical professionals and pharmacist?

Medical Error Safety Checklist for Patients

☐ Am I prepared for each doctor with copies of pertinent medical records, health summary, list of medications, list of symptoms, etc.?

☐ Do I have a list of questions?

☐ Did I research my diagnosis?

☐ Did I ask my doctor if there could be other possible diagnoses?

☐ Do I know my family history?

☐ Do I need to get a second opinion?

☐ Did I follow up on my test results?

☐ Did I ask what my test results mean?

☐ Did I ask for my tests to be repeated?

☐ Do I need to find a doctor affiliated with a highly respected medical school?

☐ Have I enlisted support from loved ones?

☐ Do I need an advocate?

From *The Take-Charge Patient*, www.thetakechargepatient.com

Hospital Safety Checklist for Patients

☐   Do I have an advocate?

☐   Do I have my patient safety checklist?

☐   Did I create my list of medications and their dosages, over-the-counter medications, herbs and supplements? Have I included my allergies to medications?

☐   Did I list new medications the doctors prescribed?

☐   Do I know who my primary nurses are? Have I written down their names?

☐   Is my advocate willing to be with me during doctors' rounds?

☐   Did I create a list of questions for the doctors and primary nurses?

☐   Did I get extra help for weekends, nights and holidays?

☐   Do I have a notebook for me and my advocate to take notes in?

☐   Do I understand my diagnosis and treatment plan?

Patient Safety Checklist

Repeat each item below at each new medical encounter while you're a patient in the hospital

☐   Your full name

☐   Your date of birth

☐   Your physician's name

☐   Your diagnosis

Questions to Ask Before You Select a New Doctor

☐ Does the doctor take my health insurance or Medicare, etc.?

☐ Is the doctor board certified in her specialty?

☐ Is the doctor affiliated with the hospital of my choice?

☐ How many patients does the doctor see in a day?

☐ How long do patients have to wait in the waiting room before their appointments?

☐ How long does it usually take to get a routine appointment?

☐ How long does it take to get a sick appointment?

☐ Will the doctor fit me in if I really need to see her?

☐ How much time does the doctor usually spend with a patient?

☐ (If you are into alternative medicine.) Is the doctor involved with or open to alternative medicine?

☐ Is the doctor's practice affiliated with an urgent care center?

☐ Is the office wheelchair accessible?

☐ Does the doctor's practice use a website for appointments, education or advice?

☐ Does the doctor have a nurse practitioner or physician's assistant?

Questions to Answer Before You See Your Doctor

☐ Has something changed since my last visit?

☐ When did it change?

☐ How long has it been this way?

☐ Do I have new symptoms? (See symptoms questions on next page.)

☐ Has my medication changed since my last visit?

☐ Have I seen another doctor since this visit, and if so, do I have a copy of my medical record from that visit?

☐ Did I have a test or procedure? If so, did I bring a copy of the results?

Questions to Ask Yourself about Your Symptoms

☐ When did I first begin experiencing symptoms?

☐ When do I most notice the symptoms?

☐ How severe are my symptoms?

☐ Does anything make the symptoms worse or better?

☐ Have my symptoms changed over time?

☐ Where on or in my body are the symptoms located?

☐ Is there pain related to my symptoms? (See questions on next page.)

☐ Were the symptoms or pain first triggered by a physical event?

☐ What have I tried to alleviate the symptoms?

☐ What do I think is causing my symptoms or associated pain?

Questions to Ask Yourself about Pain

☐   Where in or on my body is the pain located?

☐   On a scale of one to ten, ten being the worst, how bad is my pain?

☐   Is the pain the same all the time or does it come and go?

☐   Is it stabbing pain or a dull ache?

☐   Is the pain knife-like or does it radiate?

☐   Is the pain shooting or throbbing?

☐   Is the pain debilitating or am I able to carry on?

☐   What brings on the pain?

☐   What makes it better?

☐   When does it tend to come on? Afternoon? Evening? In the middle of the night?

☐   What have I tried to alleviate pain?

Questions to Ask Yourself after You See Your Doctor

☐ Did I feel comfortable with my doctor?

☐ Did I get all my questions answered?

☐ Do I feel comfortable with the diagnosis she gave me? Do I agree with the doctor's diagnosis and treatment plan?

☐ Do I understand what the doctor told me?

☐ Do I understand what the doctor wants me to do?

☐ If I received a prescription for a medication, do I know what the name of the medication is, what it is for and when I am supposed to take it?

☐ If I am to have a procedure, do I know the name of the procedure, what it is, what it is for, what I need to do to prepare for it and what I need to do following the procedure?

Ask yourself, do I feel comfortable following the doctor's recommendations? Do I need a second opinion?

Questions to Ask Your Doctor about Your Diagnosis

☐   What is my diagnosis?

☐   Where can I find information about my diagnosis? Do you have information you can give me?

☐   Are there any other possible diagnoses for my condition?

☐   What do I need to do to recover?

☐   How long do you think it will take for me to recover?

☐   What tests and procedures do I need to have done?

☐   Are there alternatives to tests and procedures?

☐   What changes do I need to make to support my recovery?

☐   Do I need another appointment with you?

Ask yourself, do I feel comfortable with my diagnosis or do I need a second opinion?

Questions to Ask Your Doctor about Your Treatment Plan

☐ What does the treatment consist of?

☐ What will I have to do?

☐ How long will it take and how often will I receive treatment?

☐ What are the side effects? Are any long lasting or permanent?

☐ Will I need extra care at home?

☐ Will I be able to work?

☐ What are the costs of this treatment?

☐ Will my health insurance cover the cost?

Ask yourself, do I feel comfortable with my treatment plan or do I need a second opinion?

Questions to Ask Your Doctor about Tests and Procedures

☐   What is the procedure/test?

☐   What are you looking for?

☐   How long will it take?

☐   Do I have to prepare for this procedure/test?

☐   What are the risks and benefits to this test?

☐   Are there any side effects?

☐   Is this test covered by my health insurance?

☐   Will I be able to drive home after this test?

☐   Do I need to have someone drive me to the test?

☐   Will I be able to go back to work right after?

☐   Will there be pain or discomfort with the test?

☐   When can I get the results of the test?

Ask yourself, do I feel comfortable with having this test or procedure or do I need a second opinion?

Questions to Ask Your Doctor about a Surgery

- ☐ What is the surgery you want to perform?

- ☐ Is your fee covered by my health insurance?

- ☐ Is the hospital or surgery center covered by my health insurance?

- ☐ Is the anesthesiologist's fee covered by my insurance?

- ☐ Do you have informational materials you can give me about this type of surgery?

- ☐ How many of these surgeries have you performed? What is your success rate?

- ☐ Would you mind if I talk to one or two of your other patients who had this surgery?

- ☐ What will the surgery do for me?

- ☐ What happens if the surgery is not successful?

- ☐ What are the risks to this type of surgery?

- ☐ Will the surgery be performed in the hospital or in a surgery center?

- ☐ What will my recovery be like? Please describe my after-care.

- ☐ Will I be in pain after the surgery?

- ☐ Will I need someone to help with my care after the surgery?

Ask yourself, do I feel comfortable with having this surgery or do I need a second opinion?

From *The Take-Charge Patient*, www.thetakechargepatient.com

Questions to Ask about Medications

- ☐ What is the name of the medication you prescribed for me? (Ask for both brand and generic names.)

- ☐ Does it matter whether I take the brand-name or generic version of this medication?

- ☐ What is the dosage and how many times a day do I need to take it?

- ☐ How long will I be on the medication?

- ☐ Why am I taking this medication?

- ☐ Do I need to take this medication with or without food or at any particular time of day?

- ☐ Are there any side effects to this medication?

- ☐ How long do you want me to take this medication?

- ☐ Can this medication interact with any of my other medications?

Questions to Ask Your Pharmacist

☐ I'm confused about all the medications I'm taking. Can you please go over them with me?

☐ What is each medication for?

☐ Which are brand and which are generic?

☐ Do any of my medications cause serious side effects? What are they?

☐ Are there alternatives to some of my medications that don't cause these side effects?

☐ I don't remember exactly when I'm supposed to take my medications. Can you give me guidance?

☐ Should I take any of my medications with food or on an empty stomach?

☐ I also use another pharmacy to fill some precriptions. Can you add those medications to your computer system?

☐ Do you have an up-to-date list of my medication allergies?

☐ I also take (list over-the-counter medications and supplements). Do any of them interact with prescription medications I'm taking?

☐ Can you give me some ideas on how to keep track of my medications?

Questions to Ask about Your Health Insurance Provider

☐   What is my co-pay?

☐   What is my deductible?

☐   Which doctors does my insurance plan allow me to see?

☐   Which hospitals, clinics or surgery centers does my insurance plan allow me to use?

☐   Am I seeing in-network providers? If not, how much will an out-of-network provider cost? Will my health insurance plan pay anything if I see a doctor who does not take insurance?

☐   Does my plan cover prescription medications?

☐   Does my health insurance cover nurse practitioners and physician's assistants?

☐   Does my plan cover acupuncture, physical therapy and other therapies?

☐   Does my plan cover me if I travel outside of the United States?

If I have primary and secondary insurance, do I understand what each one covers?

Questions to Ask If You Are Diagnosed with a Serious Disease or Chronic Medical Condition

☐ Can you describe my disease or medical conditon?

☐ What are the causes of my disease or medical condition?

☐ What are the most successful treatments for my disease or medical conditiion?

☐ What are the side effects of the treatment?

☐ What is the success rate of the treatment?

☐ Is there a consensus about medical treatment?

☐ Are there alternative treatments?

☐ Can you help me understand why this is the best treatment for me?

☐ Who will be in charge of my treatment?

☐ Do I need to see additional doctors?

☐ If this were your diagnosis, what would you do next?

☐ What else can I do to support the medical treatment?

Ask yourself, do I feel comfortable with the proposed treatment or do I need a second opinion?

From *The Take-Charge Patient*, www.thetakechargepatient.com

Index

About Martine Ehrenclou

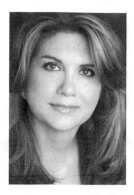

Martine Ehrenclou is an author, patient advocate and speaker. Author of the multiple award-winning *Critical Conditions* and her newest health book, *The Take-Charge Patient*, Martine is focused on empowering patients so they become experts on how to take charge of their medical care. Her mission is to bring to light the importance of being an advocate for others and for ourselves. Through her books, published articles, media interviews, blog, and lectures, Martine reveals the importance of collaboration and partnership between patients and medical professionals as well as how to navigate the health care system.

Six months into her research for *The Take-Charge Patient*, Martine developed debilitating, chronic pain and used every strategy in this book. She went from an advocate for others to an advocate for herself, and became her own take-charge patient. After eleven doctors failed to diagnose her correctly, Martine found her own diagnosis and the exact surgeon to treat her successfully. She is now pain free.

Martine writes monthly articles for several health websites, regularly publishes articles on the topics of patient empowerment, patient advocacy, patient safety and other health/medical related issues. She is interviewed regularly on national TV, radio, newspapers and magazines, including ABC News, *Woman's Day*, *Family Circle*, *Los Angeles Times Magazine*, the *Los Angeles Times*, *Publishers Weekly*, and many more. Martine also lectures at universities, hospitals, organizations and libraries, and writes a monthly blog.

Martine earned a master's degree in psychology from Pepperdine University. She lives in Los Angeles with her husband and daughter.

Visit her website at www.thetakechargepatient.com.